"In this powerful collection of stories, Carlamay Sheremata masterfully captures the complex experiences of youth, offering profound insights into what helps them feel safe enough to open up to adults. These stories were moving and emotionally impactful but also serve as a crucial reminder of the importance of fostering strong, supportive relationships with our youth. As a parent, I found myself deeply moved by these narratives, which underscore the vital role we play in helping our children navigate their formative years. The writing is accessible, making this book an invaluable resource for parents, educators, and anyone involved in supporting youths. It is equally beneficial for youth themselves, providing a meaningful opportunity for shared reading and discussion with their parents.

This book highlights the essential need for at least one trusted adult in a youth's life—a person who can make all the difference in helping them feel heard, valued, building up their inner resilient in the face of challenges. It's a poignant reminder of how such connections not only support their emotional well-being but also reveal their own abilities and strengths.

I recommend this book for anyone committed to understanding and nurturing the next generation."

–Chantal Côté Registered Psychologist
Helping Teen Girls Build Unbreakable Mindsets

"Youth today face a complex web of challenges that extend far beyond the classroom. Drawing from over eight years of experience as a School Resource Officer, Carlamay Sheremata provides a deeply insightful look into the myriad issues confronting our young people today. From the relentless pressures of academic expectations and cyberbullying to the impact of troubled home environments and the pervasive influence of social media, Sheremata offers a compassionate and authentic portrayal of the struggles that youth face daily. This book is a vital resource, offering not just a stark illumination of these problems, but also practical guidance on fostering supportive and understanding environments for our youth. By weaving personal anecdotes with professional insights, She inspires us to take collective action to nurture, support, and empower the next generation, reminding us that with grace, love, and the right tools, our youth can indeed emerge resilient and brilliant."

–Connie Jakab

YOUTH
TRUTH

Carrie

All the Best!

YOUTH TRUTH

Engaging in
Conversations
That Can
Change Lives

CARLAMAY SHEREMATA

ISBN (paperback): 978-1-0689986-2-1
ISBN (ebook): 978-1-0689986-3-8
ISBN (audio): 978-1-0689986-0-7

Book design and production by www.AuthorSuccess.com
Cover art by Adobe Stock

Printed in the United States of America

Note to the Reader

Thank you for taking the time to read my book. As you read each chapter, select content may contain material that can be triggering or disturbing to some readers, particularly those who have experienced bullying, suicide, eating disorders, mental health-related traumas, etc. If any of the material is triggering or distressing, please seek support from a trusted family member, friend, or professional.

Explicit material is included so that you, the reader, feel that you can understand the pain and emotions of the young people involved, and know that you can be a strong support and anchor for the hurting youth in your life.

Contents

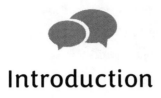

Introduction

Youth today face a multitude of challenges, both in their school environments and everyday lives. As a former police officer, I spent eight and a half years as a School Resource Officer (SRO) inside the high schools, where I was deeply immersed with both staff and students. Through this journey, I witnessed firsthand the struggles that youth face on a daily basis—not only at school but also at home. Each student brings their home life into the classroom, carrying the weight of their personal experiences on their shoulders.

The landscape of youth challenges has evolved significantly over the years. When I first began my tenure as a School Resource Officer, the issues were more contained and limited to certain periods of the day when students were at school or in their neighborhoods. However, with the advent of technology, these issues expanded into a relentless, 24/7 cycle. Social media, instant messaging, and other digital platforms have created an environment where the pressures and anxieties that youth face never truly end.

There are Challenges in Schools

In schools, students grapple with a variety of pressures. Academic expectations are higher than ever. Students are being pushed to achieve excellence in their studies, often at the expense of their mental health. Bullying, both physical and cyber, remains a pervasive issue, causing immense stress and anxiety. Peer pressure to fit in, to excel, and to conform to societal standards can be overwhelming. Many students feel isolated and misunderstood, struggling to find their place and identity amidst the chaos.

The transition from traditional bullying to cyberbullying has had a profound impact on students. Bullying no longer ends when the school day does; it follows them home through their phones and computers. The anonymity of the internet often emboldens bullies, making their attacks more vicious and persistent. This constant barrage can lead to severe consequences, including anxiety, depression, and in extreme cases, suicidal thoughts.

There are Challenges at Home

Home life for many students is another battleground. Family dynamics can range from supportive to highly dysfunctional. Some students deal with domestic violence, substance abuse, financial instability, or neglect at home. These issues compound the stress and emotional turmoil they experience, making it difficult for them to focus on their education or personal growth.

The effects of a troubled home life are often visible in the classroom. Students may exhibit behavioral problems, struggle with academic performance, or withdraw socially. Teachers and school staff, despite their best efforts, can find it challenging to provide the level of support needed to help these students thrive. The weight of their home lives hinders their ability to fully engage in their education and develop healthy relationships with peers.

There is the Role of Technology

As technology has become more integrated into our daily lives, its impact on youth cannot be overstated. Social media platforms, while offering opportunities for connection and expression, also serve as arenas for cyberbullying and unrealistic comparisons. Students are constantly bombarded with images and messages that shape their perceptions of themselves and their world. The pressure to curate a perfect online persona adds another layer of stress, contributing to feelings of inadequacy and self-doubt.

The omnipresence of technology means that students are rarely able to escape these pressures. Notifications, messages, and social media updates can intrude on their lives at any moment, disrupting their ability to relax and disconnect. This continuous connectivity has led to an increase in anxiety and sleep disorders among youth, further affecting their overall well-being.

There is the Growing Need for Support

As I observed these issues unfold, I noticed a troubling trend: youth were becoming more secretive and withdrawing into themselves. The burden of their struggles often felt too heavy to share, leading to a sense of isolation and helplessness. My heart ached for these students, who so desperately needed an outlet to express themselves and find support.

The need for a safe space where youth can be themselves, free from judgment and pressure, is more critical than ever. Schools and communities must work together to create environments that foster open communication, emotional support, and genuine understanding. Providing resources such as counseling, peer support groups, and mental health education can help students navigate their challenges more effectively.

Throughout my years as a School Resource Officer, I have seen the resilience and strength that youth possess. Despite the immense challenges they face, they have the potential to overcome adversity and achieve great things. It is our responsibility to support them; to listen to them with grace, love, and compassion; and to provide them with the tools they need to succeed.

This book leads us all on a journey to delve deeper into these issues. I share stories and insights from my own experiences in the trenches with both staff and students. My hope is to shed light on the realities of the struggles that our youth are facing in this modern world and to inspire a collective effort to empower and uplift the next generation. By acknowledging their voices and addressing their needs, we can help our youth shine brightly, like diamonds emerging from the rough.

CHAPTER I

Firestarter:
Trapped in the Shadows
of Desperation

Jon's story

Have you ever had that feeling of exhaustion, and you can finally lay your head on the pillow and then everything changes in an instant?

It had been a very long day. I was finally able to crawl into bed around 11:30 p.m. and as my head hit the pillow, my phone went off. I looked at the number and was not sure who it was, as I did not recognize the number. I was so tired and really did not want to answer the call, but my gut told me to take it. On the other side of the phone was a very calm voice; a voice I recognized but could not put my finger on a name. This voice said, "This is Jon. I am not sure if you remember who I am, but I need you . . . now."

At that moment, time stood still. The way that Jon spoke those words left a very uneasy feeling that came over my body. You know that feeling when something is just not right, and you are preparing yourself for what is to come? "Hi, Jon," I said. "Yes, I do remember you. Are you doing okay?" At least with this simple question, I would still get an answer. Jon replied, "Not good. I really need to talk to you. I am at the end of my rope, and I have no more give. No one understands me, who I am, what I am going through and what I need. No one has even asked." My heart sank, and I could feel his pain coming through the phone. I asked Jon, "What do you need from me right now?" Jon began to cry and through his sobs I heard the words "gasoline" and "ready to end it all." I immediately jumped out of bed, still holding the phone to my ear, and asked Jon to repeat what he had just said. Jon repeated his words, "I have doused myself and the living room in gasoline, and I am holding a lighter ready to end it all. I need to talk with you. Please do not send any other cops here, because if it's not you, I will flick the lighter and be done." My mind began racing and my heart began to beat faster and faster. I felt at that moment that if I did not get to him immediately, we would be dealing with a very tragic incident. I informed Jon that I would immediately be on the way to him. I got his address, and asked him to please not set himself on fire, that there was so much more for him and he had a purpose.

Jon was a sixteen-year-old young man who kept very much to himself. I would see him wandering up and down the halls of the high school every so often and would say hi to him, but he never caused problems or ever posed a concern . . . or so I thought. He had dated a few girls that I knew about, who also kept to themselves. The one thing I did notice more recently was how gaunt his face was beginning to look. His skin had a slight yellowish color, and his clothes were becoming a lot baggier. I started wondering if he was eating, and if not, what the reason might be. I touched base with a few of his teachers to ask them if they had noticed anything off, and a couple said that they had, but they never checked with him or asked other staff about it. No parents ever attended parent-teacher conferences, and there had been no communication with a parent since the beginning of classes.

As I was getting dressed, I contacted the street sergeant for the area Jon lived in and asked him to please find me two constables (police officers) who were very good at dealing with youth, as we all know that not everyone has the empathy and compassion for youth and what their struggles are. He was on it, and I let him know I was on my way to the residence, and if the constables could contact me once they were selected. I headed out the door dressed in civilian clothes (as my uniform was at the district office), jumped in the car, and made my way towards the address. I received the call from the constables that had been selected and updated them with the information and details that were known. What the public may not know is that when a police officer is sent to a scene, the only information and details that they know is what was given to the 911 dispatch from the caller. Many times, the information that a constable is informed of will lack important details. Therefore, a constable may not be fully aware of what they are heading into in many instances. I told the constables that I would meet them at the residence. Upon arrival, the fire department, emergency services (EMS), and police were there waiting on the sidewalk for me. The strong smell of gasoline was lingering in the air. This feeling of pain came over my entire body; we were in a life-or-death situation. I called Jon back and he answered. I let him know I was outside his residence with fire and EMS for precautionary reasons and asked how he was doing. Jon replied, "Constable S, I am so sorry that it has gotten to this level. I do not want to cause any more pain to anyone or be a pain in the ass. So many people would be better off if I was not around anymore." "Jon, what happened that got you to this place?" I inquired. I was thinking back to the last number of times that I had encountered him in the halls, stopped and chatted with him, but maybe that had not been enough. Maybe I had missed what was really going on. I loved my job, and especially loved the fact that each day I had the amazing opportunity to connect with these youth, see what made them tick, and find out who they really were. Did I miss something about Jon that may have been right in front of my eyes?

The phone went silent for a few seconds, and then, with his voice quivering, Jon began to tell me his story:

> *Constable S, I know you all want me to come outside but I really need to tell you something. I have never told anyone what I am about to tell you, as I am so embarrassed and ashamed. When I stop and think about this, I want to believe it's just a dream, yet when I walk through my front door each day, this is no dream. It's my re-occurring nightmare that never seems to end. Each morning as I open my eyes, I look around my room. My room consists of a mattress on the floor; a mattress that has springs popping out of it. I don't even know what a good night's sleep feels like as every time I move, I get woken up by a spring poking into my back. Once I crawl off the mattress, I think about looking outside of the window and feeling the bright sun's heat on my face. Instead, if the window is not covered by a towel, when I look out, I see a parking lot and no sun ever, as it is hidden by the concrete buildings. How I wish I could feel the warmth of the sun. If I close my eyes, I can actually feel what that would be like. I get dressed into one of the three pairs of pants I own, grab one of the three T-shirts I own; there are so many holes in the shirts that I must wear a coat over the top, even if it is hot outside. My shoes can literally talk themselves, as the soles are coming apart from the fabric and I keep having to duct tape them*

closed. I head down the hall to check on my mom. I need to make sure she got home safely. You see, my mom is a stripper and works nights. Constable S, there are so many nights I lay awake waiting to hear the key turn in the lock so I know my mom made it home safe. I can't even imagine what I would do without her. I love her so much and wish she did not have to do that job. That is not who she is, yet she feels that is all she is worth. Once I know Mom is safe and does not have any new bruises or cuts to her face and body, I head to the kitchen. I cannot remember the last time there was food in the fridge or cupboards. Some days, when I sit at the kitchen table, I close my eyes and imagine what a homemade waffle with maple syrup, fresh berries, and whipped cream would taste like. I would savor that taste forever if I could. I tell my stomach to stop making the sounds, pack my school bag, and head to school. I have an older brother, but he is in jail. I also have a dad. I have only met him twice, as he is also in jail. Mom says they will get out one of these days. She has been saying that for the past four years. I just nod at her. I know you have seen me at school early, and I remember you asking me why I come so early. The truth is that I don't want to be at home, as it is very depressing, and for me, school is a safe place.

I know I don't have a lot of friends, but I know that I am okay there. Do you remember the day you stopped me in the hall and gave me a cafeteria card so that I could eat lunch for that week? I asked you, "Why me?'" and you said to me that something inside you told you that I needed food. Constable S, the truth is that I had not eaten in four days. When you stopped me that morning, I felt like you were my guardian angel. I took the card, turned away, and *had tears streaming down my face. No one had ever done anything like that for me before. No one knows my life; no one has ever asked me if I am okay or if I need anything. I probably would not let them know the truth, but just being asked would let me know that I am worth something and that someone cares. Today, when I got home from school, I walked in the door, and there was Mom. She was sitting on the couch beaten up, with a bloody face and bruising on her arms, legs, and stomach. She said she could not go back to work as she was afraid of getting killed. But guess what? She knew that if she did not work, we would be kicked out of our place and be homeless, so off she went. I sat there for a long time. I figured that if I was not around, my mom would not feel like she had to work, and she could start a new life. That's when I thought about lighting myself on fire.*

I could not believe what I had just been told. I had tears rolling down both cheeks and as I pulled the phone away from my ear, I heard an ever-so-faint I'm sorry coming from the other side of the phone. I looked over at the sergeant and the two constables who were standing near the house and just shook my head. How could it have gotten to this point? I took a few moments to get myself together and then asked the sergeant along with Fire and EMS if I could call Jon out of the house, and if everyone was ready for whatever was to come next. There was a "thumbs-up" all around, so I called out to Jon first to see if he could hear me. "Jon, can you clearly hear my voice?" Jon answered that he could. I then continued with the commands, "Jon, slowly make your way toward the door keeping both hands up in the air. Please do not make any sudden movements. Once you step outside the door, stop." Jon followed my commands, and once outside the door he stopped. Jon looked up and I could see his face lit up by all the emergency lights. He looked towards where I was standing and a small smile came across his face and he said, "Hi, Constable S. Thank you for saving me. You are my angel."

Suddenly, his body twitched, and it looked like an enormous weight had just been taken off him. He asked if he could bend down and put the lighter on the ground, and I told him he could. Jon bent forward and placed the lighter on the ground next to his feet. I continued to give him directions: "Jon, walk five steps towards me and stop. Jon, place both hands behind your head with fingers locking together. Jon, please go into a kneeling position on both knees." Jon obeyed the commands. By this time, both Fire and police had slowly made their way toward Jon. He was asked if he had anything sharp on his body, and a quick pat down was conducted to ensure the constables were safe and Jon was safe. I walked over to him as he was being helped up, his body and clothing drenched in gasoline, looked into his teary eyes, and with a shaky voice I said to him, "Jon, you are worth so much more than you tell yourself. I believe that there is a reason that you did not flick the lighter tonight. You have a purpose on this Earth, and you have not yet fulfilled what it is." I could not contain my tears anymore. I turned around and just let the tears flow. He had an angel surrounding him that night. He saw me as his angel, yet I knew there was one overlooking everything. As Jon was being led to the ambulance, I asked one of the firefighters if it was safe for me to have a look at the scene inside the house. He said that I could go in.

I walked up to the open front door of Jon's home and walked in. The strong smell of gasoline was nauseating. As I looked around the room, I noticed the couch, area rug, and curtains were all wet from the gasoline, and in the middle of the living room stood the empty can. I stopped and closed my eyes. To think that with one flick of the lighter, lives could have been changed forever that night. I walked over into the kitchen and up the stairs to the second floor. To the right I came upon Jon's room. It was exactly how he had described it to me, mattress, clothes, and all. My heart ached for this young man. I turned and walked back down the stairs and out of the house. I made my way to the ambulance where Jon was being checked over. He asked if I could come along, as they were going to transport him to the hospital. I asked the sergeant on scene, and he agreed. I sat down beside Jon in the ambulance, and we headed to the hospital. Jon just stared at me. "Constable S, I will never be able to thank you enough for hearing my cry for help and coming to save me. I will be forever grateful to you." He held out his hand to me and I took it. At that moment, I saw my own child lying there, crying out for help. I could not help but put aside the being a cop part and just be a mom. This young teen needed me right now and I was exactly in that position . . . exactly where I needed to be right at that moment.

At that moment, I thought how many of us as parents, teachers, grandparents, or caregivers to youth have been in that right moment at that right time, and yet we pass it along as if it's nothing. To someone in a world of hurt and pain, that moment could be a life and death moment, and we may be that guardian angel. We do not know what others are facing or going through, and even if we did, no two situations are ever the same. So, remember that no matter how busy you are, it's important to always take the time to check in. As a parent, a teacher, or a caregiver of a youth, we all are busy and there are never enough hours in the day. However, the importance of a check in can be priceless.

I've also learned that it is important that we go with our gut. Each of us is given this "sixth sense," as some call, it or even a "Spidey sense," but how many of us actually listen to it and then go with it? Paying attention to that one gut feeling can change a life forever.

CHAPTER 2

You Can Run but You Can't Hide: Running from the Shadows of Substance Abuse

Jane's Story

We all have that one kid who, no matter what you tell them, because you are the parent, it goes in one ear and out the other. Yet, when the same thing is said by someone other than their parent, it's OMG it is the best advice EVER!!!!!!

There she was, slumped in a chair in my office at the school. I am not sure how she got in there, but that was beside the point. Jane was a fifteen-year-old, tenth grader who had been missing in action (MIA) for the past five days. She often vanished for days at a time and indulged in substance abuse. Her substances of choice were crack, meth, and alcohol. As I walked into my office, the strong aroma of stale smoke and alcohol was so potent that it actually caused me to gag. I nearly tripped over her bag that she had left near the door, a half-empty bottle of vodka sticking out the top. Jane looked like she had not slept in days, looking extremely tired and haggard. She looked up at me and with eyes that could not focus said, "I am sorry for the stench. I had nowhere else I could go, and I knew that you would not turn me away. I have been binging non-stop for the past four days and have hit rock bottom. I'm not sure even what day it is, but I just knew I was safe here." I nudged the door open far enough that we could continue our conversation in private, but that I could still get some fresh air circulating. The smell was bad.

I had known Jane for almost a year at this point. She had first come to my attention when she was in grade nine. I had attended the junior high school that she was at on a call for an assault that had occurred. Several girls had gotten into a fight over one of them messing with the other's boyfriend. At the time of that event, Jane had been intoxicated and was the instigator of that fight, so I had my hands full. I ended up driving her home and having a meeting with her parents. She came from a loving home where both parents were feeling torn as they felt compelled to give tough love but did not want Jane to take off and not come back. They were both at their wit's end. Jane's mom took her up to her room while I sat with her dad. He began to tell me about the continuous struggles they experienced with Jane the previous year, everything they had done to help her, even paying out of pocket for testing through a psychologist to find out what all was happening with their once so loving and kind-hearted daughter. He broke down in tears, looked at me, and asked, "Where did I go wrong?" This was not the first time I had heard this from a parent in crisis: parents feeling that they had done all they could with what they knew, yet never feeling it was enough.

Jane's mom was making her way down the stairs and as she sat down, tears were streaming down her face. Her husband placed his hand on her back and pulled her in close. The pain that these two were feeling for their child was heartbreaking to watch. I could feel the love that they had not only for each other but also for their daughter. They needed guidance and support from anyone who could help them. As I sat and listened, I began to think about what I would do as a parent if this was my child; who would I reach out to and feel safe enough to speak with? I asked them if they had contacted any rehabilitation organizations, and they said that they had contacted two of them. They were both very expensive, but their daughter was priceless, and they were going to figure out how they could come up with the funds. After brainstorming a bit more with Jane's parents, an action plan was put into place which included the next steps that needed to happen. I planned to return the following week and help them with transporting Jane, if needed, once all arrangements were in place. As I got up to leave, Jane's mom jumped up and ran over and hugged me. "No one has taken the time out like this for us and our daughter. Words cannot express how thankful we are." I felt a sense of relief come through her body as she hugged me. I knew that if this was my child, I would hope that someone would be there for me.

I received a call five days later from Jane's mom, informing me that they had secured the funds for rehabilitation for Jane and a bed was available for her. Next would be the tough part: breaking the news to Jane. Her mom asked if I would come to the house and sit with them as they chatted with her. I asked her if she wanted me in uniform or in plain clothes. She said it did not matter, so I went over in uniform since I was working. Once I arrived at the house, I went to the door and knocked. Jane answered the door and gave me a big hug. She told me she knew why I was there and that she was ready to go. I was a bit taken aback but felt a sense of relief that there would be no resistance. Jane had her suitcase ready, gave her

Mom and Dad a hug, and said that she would like me to drive her. I looked back at her parents, and I could see little smiles on each of their faces along with a look of relief. Her parents would follow behind in their own vehicle. We were off to rehab.

Once in the car, Jane started to talk. I was a bit surprised, as I had only talked with her once before, but I was glad that she felt safe and comfortable talking to me. She started out first by asking me if I had any kids. I told her I did; I had a son who was two at the time. She then continued talking:

> *You know, I often wonder if my parents ever thought that their eldest child would be in this position. As a parent, do you ever think about that? Will my child be an addict? I don't know if I would ever think that. My parents have been such amazing parents, supportive and loving, and I know have tried their best with me. I just hate rules and I don't need anyone telling me what I can and cannot do. My friends are so lucky; their parents let them hang out with whoever they want and have no curfew. My parents want to know who my friends are, who I am talking to on my phone, and I have a curfew. It sucks. What do you think, constable?*

I looked in my rearview mirror at her, and as I did, I saw such a young little girl, trying so hard to be an adult, yet she was still just a child. "Jane," I said, "As I listen to you, I remember when I was your age and how I wished that my parents were like my friends' parents. Now when I look back, I am so glad they were the way they were, like how your parents are. I am glad that they cared about who I hung out with, and where I was, and they had rules even when I did not agree with them. Your parents love you and are trying so hard to show you in these ways. I know it's hard to see that right now. Jane, I am very proud of you for agreeing to attend this program. This decision took a lot of guts to agree to on your part and know it does not go unnoticed." I looked back again in the rearview mirror and noticed Jane wiping away tears. This precious child was so lost and yearning to find where she belonged. For the remainder of the trip we drove in silence. Once we arrived at the center, I opened the door for Jane because in police cars, the back door can only be opened from the outside, and as she got out, she looked around to see if her parents had arrived. As they pulled up into the parking lot, Jane went around to the passenger side and opened the door for her mom. She helped her mom out, and as she did, Jane gave her mom a big hug and said "thank you" to her. Her mom's eyes filled with tears. A worker approached us from the center and spoke briefly with Jane's parents. Jane's mom motioned to Jane to follow them inside. Jane ran over to me and gave me a hug that I would never forget and followed the worker inside. As I turned, Jane's mom yelled out to me, "Thank you so much for believing in our daughter. We will never forget this." I opened the door to my police car, and as I did, I said a little prayer for protection over Jane and whatever was to come her way.

Little did I know that I would be seeing her again so soon. Now, in my office sat Jane, hung over and coming down from the last four days of being high. What had happened to the girl I drove to rehab? Was this the same one? I asked her if her parents knew that she was safe. She had not let them know yet but asked me if I could contact them. I made a quick call to her mom and let her know that Jane was in my office and safe. I asked her if it was okay if I talked with Jane to find out what had happened and asked her whether she wanted to be present. Jane's mom told me to please talk with her and that she would let us chat first before she made her way to the school. Jane gave me a "thumbs-up." I hung up the phone and looked at her. "Jane, what happened? The last time I saw you, you were walking into rehab." Jane pulled her knees up to her chest like in a sitting fetal position, looked up at me and said:

Well, I lasted two weeks in rehab then I got into a fight with one of the other residents and took off that night. There was no way that I was going back since I knew I would be in trouble with my supervisor. I called my parents and let them know what had happened, and they came and got me. However, they told me that I had to go back to the center and tell them myself that I would not be returning. So, I did. Once I was free from that place, my parents said that if I was to be living under their roof again, I would have to follow some strict rules like an early curfew, home right after school to do homework on weekdays, and my phone privileges would be taken away.

What the hell was this? I felt like I was back in rehab with these rules. So, I contacted one of my friends and said I needed a place to stay until I figured stuff out. I took off from home, and for the next two months, I lived between the shelters and the street. Every so often I would contact my parents to let them know I was alive, but that was all I would give them. I did not need the lectures and nagging from them. I attended school when I wanted to and was just able to barely pass grade nine. During the summer I went back home, and mom and dad were so afraid of me leaving again that they kept the rules very minimal. That was fine by me. I got a job and just hung out with my friends. Grade ten started, and I found myself with a not-so-great group of people I thought were my friends. I quickly learned that they were leading me down a messy path quicker then I was ready for. I began skipping school and staying out until early hours in the morning. I was drinking most days and began using crack and meth. One day I came home when I was still high, and as I was heading upstairs to my room, my mom walked out of my room with something in her hand. She had found my stash that I had hidden, I guess not very well. That was the last straw. My mom and dad told me that enough was enough, and I had to leave the house. So, I packed a small bag with a couple of items and headed out of the house. I knew I had burned a bridge that was not going to be easy to build again.

I ended up staying with a friend at a flophouse, and things just got worse. I still came to school when I wasn't high, which became less and less, and I still had a few friends here who worried about me. One thing I always remembered was that you were here at the school, and I liked you. You got me, which was rare. Then, five days ago, I stopped by my house to see my parents, and we got into an argument and I left again. I headed to the flophouse, and for the last four days all I know is that I drank and smoked up and did not sleep. To be honest, I do not remember much. This morning when I finally came to, I looked around the room barely remembering where I was and realized that I am in trouble. I have hit rock bottom. Constable S., I need help.

At that moment I knew why I was where I was and doing what I loved to do. If it was just to be here for one troubled young woman, that was enough. I asked Jane what she wanted me to help her with right at that moment and she answered, "Take me back to rehab. I am ready!" I looked at her and double checked with her that I heard correctly that she was ready, and she said again, "I am ready!" I got up and went over to give her a hug, and Jane whispered through her tears, "Thank you for not giving up on me." I told her, "Jane, I never did, and I never will. You are a gift, and you deserve a great life. You just have to believe that you deserve it."

I contacted Jane's mom and let her know about our conversation and what the next steps would be. I then contacted the rehab center and spoke to one of the facilitators. I let them know that I would be on my way with Jane, and asked if someone would be able to meet us once we arrived. I then asked Jane to do something very tough but very necessary. I asked if she would dump out the bottle of vodka that she still had in her bag. She agreed and I followed her to the girls' washroom. She went into one of the stalls, left the door open and dumped the rest of the bottle down the toilet. That was a big step. Once back in my office, I asked her if I could go through her bag with her and if she had anything in there that I needed to know about. Jane dumped out the bag on the floor of my office and we went through what was left. There was nothing but a few items of clothes and a pack of cigarettes. She knew that the cigarettes would be confiscated once she arrived at rehab, so I told her that she could have her last one before we headed to the center. I know she was underage, and that smoking is bad for you, but I also knew that if this was the one thing that would keep her calm and that was her only ray of hope right now, I was not going to take that away from her. Once we were outside of the school, I gave her the smoke, and as she stood by the car her parents pulled up. They got out of their vehicle, walked towards Jane and the three of them hugged each other. It was the most beautiful sight. I'm glad I had sunglasses on as I could not hold back my tears. Jane's parents held her hand as they looked at her. Jane's mom said, "Jane, we love you so much and we will be here for you always. This has been one of the hardest few months of our lives, not knowing where you were. All we could do was pray that you were okay. We will be here for you once you get out of rehab and will support you however we can. We are proud of you."

Jane finished her smoke, waved to her parents, and blew them a kiss. As she got into the car, she looked over at me and said, "They are proud of me just like you told me you were, too. I got this." I placed her bag in the trunk, got into the vehicle, and drove down to the center. Once we arrived, I drove into the parking lot and noticed the same worker who had met us the previous time was waiting for us. I got out of the vehicle, opened the door for Jane, and grabbed her bag from the trunk. Jane looked at me as I handed her bag to the worker. "You know, Constable S., I believe there is a God. I know there is a heaven and a hell as I feel I have had a small glimpse of hell, and you have helped me believe that there are angels out there who can show up as good people. I believe God sent me an angel, you, to show me that no matter what, I am enough, and I am worth it and deserving. Thank you." As I gave her a hug, I noticed the worker was wiping a tear from his cheek. He gently smiled at me as he guided Jane into the center. She looked back and yelled, "See you soon." Something inside told me that this was really it. Jane was going to get the help she needed and the next time I would be here, it would be for her graduation. She did it!

So many times, as caregivers, we think that we are at the end of our ropes with our kids. We feel that no matter what we do, things won't change and then we blame ourselves. I believe that we do the best that we can with what we have, whether it be the knowledge, information, tools, or all of the above. Sometimes what we have is only what we know or have been taught, and that is okay. Continue to do the best you can and never be afraid to ask for help. Even the best of us need a tweak here and there. It's funny how we can tell our kids things, and they look at us like we have two heads, yet someone else can tell them the same thing, and it is the most amazing information ever! Oh well, one day they will understand where we are coming from. We will make mistakes, and that is okay, too. What we need to do is confess that we made a mistake and ask for forgiveness. That can go such a long way. And guess what? We are only human!

CHAPTER 3

Passion On a Plate:
A Journey of Redemption
through Cooking

Cameron's Story

Sometimes our teens think they know it best when it comes to the direction they want to go. What if they did? What could that look like, and would you be able to let them choose their own path?

It was just another day at work. Heading into the high school, I made my way to my office. I could not believe it was already November. Where had the first few months gone? As I unlocked the door, Cameron came up to me and asked if he could come by later and chat. I told him I would be available after 10:00 that morning. He thanked me and said he would see me a bit.

I had met Cameron the previous year while he was in grade nine. The principal of the junior high school had called me up to ask if I could speak with a few of the students who had been making less desirable choices. Cameron had been one of them. Cameron and his friends were known to run in a local gang that would steal cars to go for joyrides and rob other students of cell phones, runners, and even jeans (if they liked the brand). This gang-involved youth between the ages of eleven and sixteen. Cameron had never been arrested. However, that did not mean he was not participating in the criminal activity. It meant he had not been caught . . . yet. When I arrived at the junior high school, the Principal, Mr. Conrad, met me outside and pointed to a car parked directly in front of the school. He told me that he had watched the car pull up that morning, right before the bell rang, and out jumped five youth's, including Cameron. None of them had a driver's license, as they all attended the junior high school. I snickered and commented that at least they got to school on time. Mr. Conrad laughed, "Yes, you are right. I know they are stealing cars and we have had police involved before, but so many of these kids come from such messed up families and it seems that school is a safe place for them to come and be themselves. Most of these kids show up every day to school, just not the legal way." I took the license plate number down and called into our dispatch. I wanted to determine if this car was stolen, when it was reported, and who the registered owner was. Dispatch confirmed it had been stolen eight days before and sent me the registered owner's information. I let Mr. Conrad know that the boys had been using this car for the past week. I took down the names of the five kids that the principal had seen come out of it that morning, and I asked him to call them all down to the office. I was going to have a chat with each of them. I also contacted the car's registered owner to let them know it had been located and that I would be in touch regarding the process for them to pick it up. Wow, it was already a busy morning and it had just begun.

I went and had a look in the vehicle. I noticed that there was a screwdriver in the ignition, which would be used to start and stop the car. Smart. Other than that, the rest of the car was clean and had not been damaged in any way that I could see at that time. That was a blessing, as many times when stolen cars were located there was so much damage done to either inside or outside of the vehicle or both. I called dispatch to see if I could get another police unit to come and sit with the vehicle until I had met with each of the students. I headed inside to the main office, and as I walked in, all five of the boys were sitting there. No one was talking and each of them was looking down at their phone. I said hi to them and asked if I could please have each of the cell phones to keep at the front counter until after they were finished. Amazingly, they all agreed. I collected each phone and gave it to the office secretary to hold onto. I then had a quick chat with Mr. Conrad, and had the first kid, the driver, come into the principal's office. Big M, as his friends called him, was a very small blond-haired blue-eyed child who was twelve years old. He came in and sat down. I had to smile as I asked him his name. What I saw of him and what he said his name was did not match up. I asked him how he got his name. He told me he had a big attitude and people did not mess with him. Made sense. I introduced myself and then began the conversation regarding the car. "So Big M, can you tell me about that car that is parked out front of the school? I have some information that you and a few of your friends were seen in it earlier today." Big M smiled. "Well, I drove my friends to school in it this morning. I even parked it properly so I would not get a ticket." I sat there for a moment, staring at Big M. I looked over at the principal, and he was shaking his head in disbelief. Big M had told the truth. We then continued the conversation. "Big M," I said, "May I ask you where you got this car from?" He looked at me and said, "Me and a couple friends were walking down the street one evening and noticed this car parked along the road. I tried the door handle, and it was unlocked. My buddy had a screwdriver, so he stuck it in the ignition, moved it around a bit and the car started. We all jumped into the car and drove off." I sat there in awe. This kid again had told us everything. I looked at him and thanked him for being so honest. I know he could have lied or blamed someone else, but he didn't. Wow. Big M looked at me and said, "I knew as soon as I was called down to the office that I had been caught. I knew I had two choices to make: lie or tell the truth. My mom always told me that even though the truth may be hard sometimes, it's always better to tell it. Constable, I know what I did was wrong, but I have a reputation to uphold. As you can see, I am small and don't look like much of a leader. So, I must prove myself. Each day this week I picked up the boys and drove them to school. My mom would kill me if I missed class." I asked Big M, "What would your mom do if she knew you had stolen a car and had been joyriding and using it for driving your friends around?" Big M said she would be mad, and he would probably get in trouble, but it would be way less than if he missed classes. I had to laugh. Seriously, what else could I say? I asked him if he thought the others would be as honest as he was. He said he didn't know but he hoped so, and if they didn't tell the truth, he would talk with them about honesty. Again, I had to laugh. You cannot make this stuff up! I asked him to go back and sit in the main office, and as he got up, I looked at him and said, "Thank you for your honesty. I do not know many kids like you. There are still going to be consequences, but we can figure things out in a bit, okay?" He gave me a "thumbs-up," and as he left, he turned around and asked if he could give me a hug. Mr. Conrad's jaw dropped to the floor. I looked at Big M, held open my arms and received his hug. "Thank you for listening," he said.

Well, one down, four to go. Before we had the next kid come in, Mr. Conrad looked at me and said, "Carlamay, I have not seen kids open up to outsiders like this before, let alone a police officer. I am amazed. It's like you have a way with them that I have never seen before. They trust you and know they are safe talking with you. You are like the youth whisperer." Well, that was a new one! I loved working with youth and knew that many of them were misunderstood and not given a voice. Yes, there were some who used their voice in the wrong way, but if we really looked deep down, there was a reason that this was happening. My main goals with all the youth that I came into contact with was first, that each of them knew they were important, valued, and heard, and second, I was a safe place for them to land. Whether it involved talking or just hanging out, they knew that I was there for them.

Next, I went into the main office area and called Cameron in. As he walked into Mr. Conrad's office, I had him sit down. I introduced myself to him and asked him if he knew why he had been called down. He said he had an idea and he pointed out to the car in front of the school. Hmm . . . two for two. Not bad. "Cameron, can you let me know more about what's out there?" Cameron began his story:

> *That car out there is how my friends and I have been getting to school this past week. I was not there when they got the car, but after they took it, they drove over to show me. I was surprised, but also impressed. You see, I arrived in Canada two years ago from Taiwan with my mom and two brothers. My dad stayed back. When we arrived, I could barely speak or understand English, but my brothers knew a bit. My family has been involved with the gangs in East Asia since before I was born, so I knew nothing else. Within five months of coming to Canada, my brother*

was arrested for gang involvement and went to jail. My other brother and my mom continued interacting with the gang ties they had here. I found this group of friends that accepted me, and we started hanging out. I began to learn that they were involved in criminal stuff, and I knew I did not want to get too involved, but I wanted to be a part of the group. This group felt like a family. I knew riding in that car was wrong and I kind of knew we would get caught one of these days.

I asked Cameron if he would let me know who was driving, and all he told me was that I had already talked to him. I thanked Cameron for being honest and then I asked him what his mom would say if she found out about him riding around in a stolen car. Cameron told me that she would be madder about the fact that he got police involved and now his family was on their radar. I understood that and let him know that he and I would chat more later. As he got up, he turned toward me and said, "You are really easy to talk to. Thank you for listening to my story." I touched his shoulder and said, "You are so welcome. I know you each have a story and I believe each of you needs to be heard."

Mr. Conrad and I continued talking to the rest of the kids who were in the car and each one told us the truth. They knew they had done wrong, and all just wanted to be part of the group. They also knew that there were consequences for their actions, and each was open to what they were. Big M ended up getting charged, and because this had not been his first time stealing a car, he ended up getting sent to jail. He did his time and once out, came over to visit me at the high school I was working at. Crazy how I was still in his good books.

As I was sitting in my office, I noticed that it was 10:30 a.m. and heard a knock on my door. Cameron had come back to see me. I motioned for him to come in. He sure had grown since the previous year. He sat down and I closed the door. Cameron began with small talk, then he took a huge breath and started to talk.

> *Constable, I am coming to talk with you because last year you treated me with such kindness and respect, even though I did not deserve it. I felt comfortable talking with you and now I really need some guidance. As you know, my family has been involved in the gang life ever since I can remember, and that is not the direction I want to go. I know I have a lot to offer as well have a passion for food and making it beautiful. I love to cook and really wanted to join the culinary program here at the school but came in too late for this year. After I got caught last year, I have begun to look at the path that I would be going down if I continued with the criminal activities. To be honest, it is not the path I want to go down. Can you help me see what is out there that I can do?*

I looked at Cameron and right away I had an idea. There was a gentleman in the community who owned a couple of restaurants. I quickly sent him an email to see if he and I could have a conversation. I wanted to see if maybe there was a way to get Cameron involved in a restaurant, even just to start by bussing or washing dishes. I knew that once this guy could see Cameron's passion and work ethic, he would begin to move Cameron up to the next level. I let Cameron know my thoughts and what I believed he could start to achieve. I told him I was proud of him, as it took a lot of guts to not just come and see me, but also to be honest about where he was heading and that he needed to make a change. He looked away, and as he did, I caught a glimpse of him wiping his cheeks. Tears were streaming down his face. He began to cry and tried to talk in between breaths. "Constable, no one has ever told me they were proud of me. Not even my mom. Sometimes, I wondered if I ever made her happy. No matter what I tried to do, whether it was keeping my marks up or standing up for something I believed in, I was never validated, and I so wanted that from her. What you said to me today gave me hope. I am a deserving person who is worth being heard and validated. Thank you for that." I gave Cameron a big hug and told him I would let him know once I heard back from the restaurant guy. He headed off to class with a little skip in his step.

A week later, I received an email back and called Cameron down to come and see me. The boy that walked through my door was a very different one from the week before. There was a confidence that came off of him of someone who knew what they wanted and believed in himself. I let Cameron know that he had been offered a job as a prep person at the restaurant. He would get to work with food and learn about food. He would also have the opportunity to learn about cooking and work with one of the chefs. Cameron was so excited. He jumped out of the chair and began to dance around. My heart was so full of joy. One person gave him a chance to believe in himself and validated him and his whole world changed. Cameron skipped out of my office, ready to take on whatever was to come his way.

So many of us as caregivers want to give advice to our youth, whether it be about the courses they should take, the career path that is best for them, or even the job that we feel would suit them. What if we allowed our youth to follow their dreams, take the courses that they wanted to take, and pursue their passions? Sure, it may not make much money or have a high place in society, but what if it made them happy? They may not want to be the lawyer, doctor, teacher, or nurse that you had hoped they would be. Maybe they want to be an auto mechanic and run their own shop. Or become an electrician or plumber and have their own business. What would happen if we did not have people that went into those professions?

It's time to stop trying to live our dreams through our kids and let them figure out who they are and what they want to become. We need to let them be able to dream, as those dreams can become reality.

CHAPTER 4

It's Not What I Thought: Disillusionment of the First Time

Jordan's Story

As a parent, have you had that oh-so-uncomfortable conversation with your teen, the one that you hope comes way later? Let me tell you about the birds and the bees . . . that one! It's the one talk that every parent should have with their kids before they learn about the subject from friends or, worse yet, social media.

Jordan walked sheepishly into my office at the high school one Monday morning. I could tell something had happened, and as my imagination began to create scenarios, he sat down in a chair, put his chin in his hands, and stared at me. This young man looked much younger than the high school students who usually came into my office. I had never met Jordan before, nor had he stood out in the halls of such a big high school. Yet, now in front of me sat this child. He started off by telling me that I looked to be around the same age as his mom. I laughed, as I had been told this before. He then got up, closed the door, sat back down, and began to sob. Jordan looked up and asked, "Why did no one ever talk to me about how I would feel after having sex for the first time?" I looked at this child and asked him what he meant. He began his story:

I was hanging out with a couple of my friends who always seemed to get the girls. We were in this community park and there was a pathway with some bushes to the side, slightly covering the view from the path. One of my friends told me that this one girl that I liked told him she wanted to have sex with me behind the bushes. But before she would have sex, I had to sign a contract. First, I could not believe she wanted to have sex with me, but I was not sure what a contract had to do with this. So, I asked my friend if I could see the contract. He told me she had it and would show me when I met up with her.

I decided to go, and I met her near the bushes by the pathway and she showed me this piece of paper. Well, it was not a contract. It was a piece of paper that said in order for me to be allowed to have sex with her, her friend could watch from the bushes, and I had to allow her to do whatever she wanted with me. If that was not enough, if I said anything to anyone, she would deny it. I was trying to quickly put this all together in my head, except it was not the right "head" that I was thinking with. So, I signed the piece of paper, and we had sex. Constable S, I thought my first time was supposed to be something special, something I would want to remember. What happened was not what I expected or hoped for. This girl got up, pulled up her jeans, gave a "thumbs-up" to her friend, which I then noticed was not only watching, but also videoing everything. I felt so dirty at that moment. Her friend laughed and they both took off. I literally was left with my pants down.

As I was listening to Jordan, I watched his eyes ever so closely. The pain and sadness I saw in them hurt me deeply. This was not how young love was supposed to be. What had happened to the butterflies and stars in the eyes, the giddiness and that feeling of excitement? What had happened to our youth and that innocence? Jordan paused for a moment, looked up at me, and said in an ever so soft voice, "You know, I cannot even talk to my mom or dad about this stuff. They don't get me. I wish I could sit down with them, like I am with you, and feel comfortable enough to just talk. Talk about anything and everything." I asked Jordan why he did not feel comfortable talking with his parents. He continued, "I was raised in church and my parents are very religious. You know, I don't even know what that really means, being religious. All I know is that sex before marriage is wrong and I have been told that there is no place for that or even thinking about it in the house. Look what I have done, I have not just thought about it but have actually had sex." Jordan looked at me, tears streaming down his face. He placed his face in his hands and cried. Sitting there, I thought back to my own upbringing. I was raised in a Baptist church, and it was very strongly encouraged that we did not have sex until we got married. I could understand what Jordan was talking about, except I had been able to talk with my mom about sex and these hard-topic conversations. It got me thinking, how many other teens were walking the halls in the high schools dealing with these very similar feelings?

I asked Jordan what would help to make things a bit easier at this moment. He sat and thought for a moment. "I would like if both my mom and dad, you, and I were able to sit down all together and talk about all that has happened, as well as what I need from them. I am not sure what their reactions will be, but it would be easier for me having you there, even as a mediator. I often wonder if my parents ever went through things like this. Maybe I should ask them one day," he said.

Jordan and I began to figure out the best place that he felt comfortable inviting his parents to have a sit-down. Would it be in a coffee shop on neutral ground, or at the house where all parties could be themselves and show their feelings? Would it be preferable for Jordan to talk in my office, where he was comfortable, although his parents might not feel at ease? I asked Jordan to think about that and to let me know what would work for him. I wanted to make sure he felt that he had some control over this situation. I wanted him to understand that he was a courageous young man who could experience his feelings, feel safe, and decide how he wanted to approach things.

It had been a few days since the incident in the park, and as Jordan was taking some time to determine these next steps, the gates of hell were about to unleash their fury. Remember that "friend" in the bushes who had been videotaping the whole event? Well, the video was now viral. To those of you who are not up with the terms, when something goes viral, it means the content has spread rapidly and widely through the internet or social media and has gained widespread attention. I had received a message from one of the teachers, Ms. Jon, asking if she could head to my office and have a quick chat. I always loved when the teachers stopped by to chat, or even just to say "hi." I heard a knock on my office door and Ms. Jon poked her head in. I motioned her to come on in, and as she did, she closed the door behind her. At that moment, I knew there was a problem. Ms. Jon asked me how I was, then proceeded to unlock her phone to locate something. "Carlamay, I am not sure if you have seen this or are even aware of it, but it is not good at all." She turned her phone towards me and pressed play. My heart sank. It was the video of Jordan and this girl having sex in the park.

I could not believe that this had been posted for everyone to see. Tears began to fill my eyes and I looked up at Ms. Jon.

My first thought was to find Jordan and make sure he was okay. Something like this might be more than someone could handle, and Jordan was already dealing with enough. He did not need this added on. I sent a message to Jordan to come and see me as soon as he could. First things first, Jordan's mental health and safety were most important. I thanked Ms. Jon for bringing this to my attention and she left my office. I began to construct a plan. First, it was crucial to connect with the administration staff before this got out of hand. Second, connecting with the girl from the incident and her friend who had recorded the incident was imperative. I sent a message to the principal and the assistant principal to see about meeting for a brief chat. I sat back in my chair, taking a much-needed breath, when I heard a knock on the door. Jordan stuck his head in. I asked him to come in and to have a seat. His eyes met my eyes. This was going to be a very hard conversation. I began, "How have you been doing? How are things at home? I know the meeting with your parents still needs to be set up." Jordan replied, "I am doing okay. I feel each day like I am in a nightmare that I never wake up from. I also just heard from a friend that the video may have been posted online. I do not know who to believe, but if this is true, I do not know if I will be able to handle this. My parents don't even know yet and the whole world may have seen something that I wish I would have never done." I watched as Jordan's face began to change. He looked up at me and asked, "Is it true about what my friend said?" I looked at him with such pain in my eyes and answered, "It's true Jordan. I am so sorry." Jordan's face went white, as if he had seen a ghost, and he slumped out of his chair to the ground and just sobbed. At that moment I knew I needed to focus on this young hurting child. I moved over to the floor, got down on my knees, put my arms around Jordan and just held him. He did not need a lecture and be told that he should have thought about what he was doing. Instead, he needed to feel loving and supportive arms around him and to know at that moment, he was in a safe place and could just be. Holding him, I felt his body begin to collapse with every deep sob, and the strong emotion and distress that each sob contained. I could not help but cry with him, my heart feeling the pain that his body was releasing. Jordan looked up at me, and through his sobs, asked me what he should do. I looked at him, and through my tears I said to him, "I've got you."

After a few moments, I released my arms from around Jordan, and with both of us sitting on the floor, I wiped away my remaining tears and gave Jordan a Kleenex. I quickly put my thoughts together and figured out the next steps. Jordan had also wiped the remaining tears from his eyes and cheeks and looked at me. His eyes looked at me like a child looked to a parent for help, guidance, and direction. I pushed myself up off the floor, put out my hand for Jordan to grab hold of and helped him stand up. Once up, he looked at me again and asked, "What's next?" As I quickly thought of all the moving parts of this scenario, I knew that two things had to happen immediately. First, I needed to speak with both girls involved, and second, Jordan and I needed to meet with his parents. "Jordan," I said, "Let's see if your parents can head to the school to meet today, as I feel that it's time to put everything out on the table. I will be here beside you and can take the lead if you would like me to. I know this will not be easy, but it will take a big weight off of you." Jordan nodded and said, "Yes, I know you are right. I will call them right now." He started dialing the number and placed his phone on speaker. His mom answered and immediately she asked if he was alright, as he usually texted and did not call. Jordan began his ask, "Hey, Mom. Yes, I am okay. I am wondering if you and Dad would be able to come and meet me here after school along with the School Resource Officer? Something happened today, and I really want to talk to you both about it." You could hear a pin drop with the silence, and then his mom spoke with the most gentle and compassionate voice, "Jordan, Dad and I can come right now if that makes things easier. Whatever is going on we are here for you and love you." Jordan looked up at me with tears in his eyes and said, "Yes, please come now and thank you, Mom, so much." They both said goodbye and Jordan sank back into the chair as relief came over his body. He felt like things were going to be alright. I asked Jordan if he would not mind waiting outside my office, as I had to make a few other phone calls. Jordan stepped out. The next thing I had to tackle was getting in touch with both girls who had been involved with the actual incident and the videoing of the incident.

I was able to locate both girls and made my way up to their classrooms and called them outside. Once outside their classrooms, I asked each of them for their phones, which they handed over. I was hoping that they would give me permission to look on their phones because if they did not, then I would have to go another route with this investigation. The principal just happened to be walking by and so I asked him if he would escort the girls down to the main office. He agreed, and the girls followed him down. I made my way back to my office. Just as I turned the corner, I saw Jordan with his mom and dad walking towards me. I stopped and waited for them, and we all went into my office. As I greeted his parents and shook their hands, I could feel their concern for the unknown. I had the three of them sit down, closed the door, and headed to my seat. I remembered that I had the other two phones in my cargo pants pocket so I pulled them out and placed them inside my desk. I looked over at Jordan's parents and at him and could see the love and concern that they both had for Jordan. I asked Jordan if he would like to start the meeting and he nodded:

> *Mom and Dad, I want to let you know about something that has happened to me. I have asked the constable to be here with me not only as support but also someone who has been by my side throughout this whole ordeal. Constable S. has shown me that no matter what, I still matter, even when I make stupid choices. I know that our faith is very important, and I know that there have been expectations that you both have of me. This past week I ended up making a stupid choice, and now it has become a huge issue. I had sex with a girl in a park, and what I did not realize was her friend was videotaping the whole thing. If that was not bad enough, it was posted on social media and went viral. That is not the way I wanted to be known and I am so sorry.*

Jordan's parents both got out of their seats, and as they came towards Jordan, he threw himself into their arms. They held each other for a moment, then looked at me and his dad asked, "What's next?" I knew at that moment that they were ready to take on whatever was to come. I had Jordan go home with his parents and let them know I would contact them as soon as I had more information. Making sure I had both girls' phones with me, I headed to the main office. I wanted to find out from these girls what their true intentions were and what they were thinking.

As I walked into the office, both girls were sitting by the door. One of the girls broke down in tears, her face in her hands. My heart felt for this young girl, as there was most likely so much more behind her actions. Ana, the girl who was crying, and who had also recorded the whole incident, stood up and followed me into the principal's office. Jess, the one with whom Jordan had sex, slowly trailed behind. Both girls sat down; I closed the door, placed their phones on the principal's desk, and as I did both girls broke down crying. Ana started her story, "Constable S. I am so sorry I was so stupid. I was only thinking about myself and how if I did this, I would now be part of the IN group. Jess had told me that she was planning on doing this to Jordan and that if I wanted to be friends with her, I was to record it. She told me where to stand, what she was going to do, and then where to post it. I did not realize the hurt and pain and damage that this would cause. I am so, so sorry." Ana looked at Jess and began to cry harder. I passed her a Kleenex and waited a moment. I looked over at Jess, who stared back at me with eyes that were so empty. I was trying to look inside her soul, but I just saw such an emptiness. I asked Jess if she had anything to say, and she shook her head back and forth and quietly said, "No." Both girls were in pain, but both showed it in very different ways. I asked the principal to please contact both of their parents, and as I did, Jess broke down and began to cry. All I heard through her sobs was, "I am so sorry. I am going to be in so much trouble."

I was curious . . . what did Jess mean by this comment? I asked her about that, and crazy enough, her and Jordan's story was eerily familiar. Jess grew up in a Christian home where not only was sex wrong, but it was never talked about. Jess had learned about it from her friends and her older sister. This scenario seems to be more and more common even in today's day and age. Why was it so difficult to talk about this topic, and did parents realize the damage this was doing not only to the relationship with their kids, but also the dangers of their kids learning it from friends, social media, and the porn industry? These teens were being left to navigate treacherous waters with barely a lifeline.

Ana's parents showed up first, and I spoke with them along with Ana and the principal. They were very disappointed and needed to process all that had occurred and then speak more with Ana at home. Ana gave me a hug before she left and whispered to me, "I promise I will do my best to right my wrong, however long it takes." I hugged her back and gave her an extra squeeze. I knew in my heart that this was a tough lesson, but she had learned from her mistakes. Jess's parents came in next. The ambiance in the room changed, and there was no hug or checking in to make sure Jess was okay. I felt sadness for Jess, as I could feel from her that she so much just wanted her mom to hug her and tell her everything was going to be okay. Jess looked at me and started crying. I held her hand as I began to talk out the scenes that had taken place over the past few days to her parents. I also let them know my upbringing and how important I know it must be for her to stay pure as I know it was to my parents. Neither parent showed any emotion. I knew this was going to be a tough battle for Jess, but I also knew that prayer could open hearts, and at that moment that was the only positive thought I had. Her parents got up, thanked both the principal and me, and began to walk out the door. As Jess got up, she looked at me, and with tears streaming down her face said, "Thank you very much for supporting me and caring for me. I have not felt a love like that in a long time." I smiled at her and gave her a big hug, holding her tight. "Jess, you are God's masterpiece and no matter what, he loves you unconditionally." As she left the office, I could not hold back my tears. I would see this teen walking up and down the halls, looking like she had it all together, beautiful, with lots of friends, and always laughing, yet she was hurting so much. All she wanted was to feel loved, valued, and know things were going to be okay.

How many parents look down at youth today, walking around with their jeans hanging low on their hips, hoods over their heads, very rarely looking up to talk to us in our eyes, and always on their phones? We cast a judgment so quickly. When you take the time to talk to one of these youth, you find out very quickly that they so badly want to be accepted; not only by their peers, but also by the adults in their lives. They wish their parents would not judge them so quickly and instead take the time to just have a conversation. The information that you learn during those conversation times could be lifesaving. Youth need to know they can be honest about what is really going on, even if they look like they have it all together. You can't judge a book by its cover.

Take the time to talk with the youth in your life, listen to what they are saying, and hear them. You may not always agree, but for them just to know that they are heard is a huge step toward knowing they have a safe place to talk and be who they are.

CHAPTER 5

Will I Still Be Loved: Courage in Confusion and the Quest for Acceptance

Byron's Story

How would it feel if you were trying to figure out who you were, had so many questions, yet had no one you could trust to talk with? What would it be like to walk down the halls at school and feel like you were never seen and never really known?

It was a cold January morning. We had just had a heavy snowfall and it had been a slow drive to the high school. I stopped by the main office on my way to my office. As I came through the door, I noticed a young boy sitting in the chairs looking down at his phone. I said good morning as I walked by and as he looked up, he looked as if he wanted to say something, yet nothing came out of his mouth. I asked him if he was here to see someone, and he said, "Actually, I don't really know who I can talk to." I put my bag down by the counter and sat beside him. I introduced myself to him and asked him his name. He said it was Byron. I asked him what he meant by what he said. Byron began to tell me his story:

I grew up in a very conservative home. My parents were wonderful, loving, caring, and kind. I never questioned their love for me. That is until one day, when I asked them what being gay meant. I had heard this term and looked up what it really meant. I was curious. My parents would have no part of it and asked why I had even brought up that topic. Well, to be honest, I was wondering about myself. You see, I have always wondered if I am different. I have always had amazing girlfriends but have never felt romantically connected with them.

I stopped Byron at that moment and asked him if we could head to my office to continue the conversation. More students and staff were beginning to roam around the office, and I wanted to make sure Byron felt comfortable and safe since this was a courageous topic to talk about. He agreed. I grabbed my bag, and he followed me to my office down the hall. I unlocked the door and we both went inside. As he sat down, I closed the door, placed my bag by the wall, and sat down next to him. Byron continued his story:

My parents never brought up the topic again and neither did I. I decided that I would keep it to myself and maybe one day, I would have a close friend I could trust with this information. Life went on. As I made my way through high school, I learned about the GSA (Gay Straight Alliance) group in the school and thought it may be a good place to start. I attended my first meeting, and it was such a great group. I was able to be myself, and I felt safe which I had not felt for a long time. I was able to hear others' stories. I also met others who were not gay but wanted to support their friends who were gay or trying to figure themselves out. I was not alone and that was such a great feeling knowing this. Well, that was all fine and dandy, but I still had to be in a house where I could not talk to my parents about this whole thing. Each day it got harder and harder to be at home knowing that if my parents knew the truth about me, I may not have a home or family anymore. What should I do?

As Byron finished his sentence, he began to cry. It was like he was finally releasing all the pent-up hurt and anger he had been holding onto. I passed him a box of Kleenex, and as he grabbed one, he apologized for his outburst. I told him I was so proud of him and what he had just let go of. This was big stuff. He was afraid that if his parents knew that he may be gay, they might not love and accept him or would they kick him out and disown him. He had heard some awful stories from others about what had happened to them when they came out to their families. He started crying again. "Byron," I said, "let's not put the cart before the horse. If you would like, I could be a part of this conversation with your parents as a mediator-type person. Not agreeing with either side, just there as a support for you." He said that would be a great idea. I asked him to see what day and time would work best, and if the school or his house would be a better location. He needed to feel safe to be able to talk with them. He told me he would think about it and get back to me. I had been a part of a few of these conversations before. Some went really well, while others were a disaster. I remembered one family who completely disowned their child. The parents threw all of his items out of the house onto the front lawn, and they never spoke with him again. Being a parent myself, I had a hard time believing how someone could do that to their own child. What about unconditional love? We may not always agree with the choices or decisions our kids make, but they are still our children and deserve compassion, empathy, and love. I was really hoping that Byron's parents would be able to see their hurting boy for who he was, and just love on him no matter what. I guess we would just have to wait and see.

Two days later, Byron came to my office and asked if we could meet with his parents the following week here at the school. We scheduled a day and time and Byron let his parents know. I knew he was nervous, but he also wanted to get this out of the way so he could begin to live his life to the fullest. One of the things he loved was musical theatre. He had auditioned for one of the main roles for that year's school production and got it. He could sing and dance and it all seemed to come so naturally. That was another thing he wanted to tell his parents about, as he really wanted them to come and see the performance. He knew this would be a big leap, especially for his dad. His dad had been a football player and his brother had gone in that direction, as well. Here he was, the black sheep of the family. He knew where he wanted to fit in, yet he did not know how to accomplish that. I would watch Byron around the school. He was so caring and compassionate, kind and empathetic. If someone needed help, he was always there to lend a hand, and if someone was short on cash in the cafeteria, he was the first one to help cover the cost. I had never met a youth like him, and I had met thousands over the years. Byron had a strength in him that took him to the next level. Whatever came in his way, he could conquer. I knew that he was a survivor and a fighter, and that he would be able to handle whatever was going to come.

The day came and Byron's parents showed up at the school. I met them in the main office along with Byron, and we all walked to my office. I could sense that his dad was feeling a bit uncomfortable. I was hoping that would change as we started talking. Once we arrived at my office, I asked them to sit down and closed the door. I began the conversation. "Hi there. I am the SRO, Constable Sheremata. Thank you both for taking the time out of your busy schedules to come and have a conversation this afternoon. I want to create a safe space for all of you, so please let me know if there is anything you need to help to create that. I want to start off by saying I am here just as a mediator and that is all. I am here to also answer questions if needed. You have an amazing son. He is such a treasure, and it has been such a blessing getting to know him." I looked over at Byron and passed the conversation his way. I could tell he was a bit nervous, but I could also see confidence in him starting to show itself. Byron looked at both of his parents and began to have a conversation with them.

> *Mom and Dad, I am so thankful for you both. I am not in trouble, but I wanted to talk with you about something that I needed a bit of support to bring it forward. I know I am different. I always have been. More sensitive and empathetic and all that. And Dad, I know I don't play football like you had hoped I would, but I am really good at singing and dancing and actually got the lead role in our school's musical theatre production this year. I am really good.*

Byron looked my way, and I nodded in agreement. He continued:

> *I have so badly wanted to make you both proud of me and I feel like I have failed in that area. For this past year, I have been struggling with figuring out who I am and where I*

fit in when it comes to relationships. I have always had a lot of female friends, yet I have never been romantically or physically attracted to them. I also have a lot of male friends and sure, I think some are handsome, but I know how I was raised, and that I am not to go that way. What if that was who I am, a gay man? Would that be a huge issue for you guys? Would I still be loved?

I looked over at his parents' faces to see if I could figure out what they were thinking. His mom had tears in her eyes and his dad, I could tell, was trying to process what was just said. Suddenly, his mom got out of her chair, came over to Byron, grabbed his hand so he would stand up and gave him a huge hug. "We will always love you no matter what Byron. We may not always agree with things, but that will never stop us from loving you." Byron hugged his mom back and said thank you. His dad was still seated when he looked up and said, "I am a bit lost for words right now. I am just trying to process all this information. Like your mom said, we may not always agree but we will never stop loving you." I looked over at Byron and he was grinning from ear to ear. All he wanted was to be loved and accepted, and that is what his parents showed him.

It is important to recognize the courage it takes to reveal one's true self. The journey towards acceptance, both from others and oneself, is deeply personal and challenging. Remember, everyone deserves to be loved and accepted for who they are. Each journey is unique, and by living your truth, you contribute to a world where authenticity and acceptance can flourish.

CHAPTER 6

Will I Be Safe: Navigating Parenthood, Eating Disorders and Abuse

Candace's Story

How many times have we seen a teenage mom walking down the sidewalk pushing a stroller or a teen couple with a young infant in tow and have quickly cast judgement on them without ever knowing their story or what they have been or are going through? What if our assumptions only scratched the surface of their reality?

It was a crisp Tuesday morning, and the smell of fall was in the air. I had just pulled up at the high school when a young girl, not more the fifteen years old, came up to my police car. As I looked up, I noticed it was Candace, a beautiful young woman who had been through a lot. I did not recognize her, since the last time I had seen her she had just had her baby. Today, I could tell that she had been crying because her eyes were red and swollen. I opened the car door and said good morning to her and asked if she was okay. She burst into tears and answered, "No, I'm not doing okay. Can I come in and talk with you in your office?" She followed me into the school. I said good morning to the office staff and unlocked the door to my office. Once inside, I placed my bag and coffee down and motioned for Candace to come in and sit in the chair. I closed the door.

I had last seen Candace when she was eight months pregnant. She had come into my office with a black eye. The baby daddy, whom Candace was no longer with, was unhappy that she had not gotten rid of the baby as he had told her she better do it. Candace knew in her heart that she did not want and could not have an abortion. After discussing things with her parents, they both supported her having the baby and then deciding whether adoption would be the best plan. Candace was really struggling with that option though, as secretly she really wanted to keep her baby. Over the previous months, Candace and I had gotten to know each other. We had a special bond. I had stood beside her and her family through some pretty hard times and Candace knew I would be there for her. When Candace and I first met, it had been at one of the hardest points in her life. She was in an abusive relationship, and it was getting worse. She had found herself losing hope.

I came from a wonderful home with two loving parents, and I was always happy and full of life. I loved my life, to be honest. I was involved in dance and swimming and was earning scholarships. My dream was to become a full-time dancer and train at Juilliard with the best. I was working toward getting my whole tuition covered through scholar-ships. Then I met 'him,' Ron. He was seventeen years old and played sports. He was everything I thought I liked, and he told me he loved me. So here I was, a fourteen-year-old with a huge crush that began to take over my life. Well, let me rephrase that: he began to take over my life. He began to tell me who I could hang out with and who I was allowed to text. Then, he began to tell me what I could and could not wear. And next it was slowly cutting my family out of my life. If this wasn't bad enough, he began to hit me, first across the back because clothes would hide it, and then he began to punch me in the face. This became a lot harder to hide. Makeup was only able to cover so much. I began to skip school because I could not hide the marks, and I had been sitting at a 95 percent overall average. What was happening to me? My parents began receiving absence notices from the school, and when they would try to talk to me, I would shut down and shut them out. I continued with my dance classes as best I could, but because I was not showing up, I began losing my scholarships. I was falling fast and so deep. I was turning fifteen, and a friend I could still talk with bought me a birthday cake. We were out in a park with a few of Ron's friends and my one friend. As I was putting a forkful of this delicious black forest cake in my mouth, my boyfriend came over and asked if I should be eating it, as he had been noticing that I was putting on weight. ARE YOU KIDDING ME RIGHT NOW???!!! I broke down in tears, threw the cake on the ground, and buried my face in my hands as I sobbed. My friend could not believe it and yelled at him. He gave her the middle finger and turned around. That is how my eating disorder started.

I began to eat only twice a day, and when I would eat, it was an apple or some crackers and cheese or something very light. I watched as I began to see each of my ribs showing. I then noticed my clothes were getting too big and my hip bones were beginning to protrude out. When

I would look in the mirror; all I would see was a skeleton looking back at me. Who was I? What happened to the once-happy dancer with a great figure? Ron would let me know how much he loved how I looked, even though I had heard his friends tell him I looked horrible and would probably wither away to nothing. Then, one day, my mom made an appointment with our family doctor. On the day of the appointment, I went inside and could tell by how the nurses looked at me that I was not looking good. My doctor could not believe what was happening and told me that if I were not careful, I would stop getting my periods. Hmmm, I thought, did that mean that if I had sex, I would not get pregnant? Well, that could be good. Ron had been pressuring me to have sex with him because he said he loved me, but I was afraid of getting pregnant, so I told him no. Now, maybe it would be okay if I kept starving myself, as he liked what I looked like when I was this thin, and if I did not get my periods, then it would be okay to have sex. I thought I had it all together and a great plan was set. What I failed to think about was not whether you could get pregnant but that all it would take was one time. And I guess God has a sense of humor because, guess what? The first time and boom . . . I was pregnant. I could not believe it! What was I going to do with a child? I was just a child myself, and there was no way I could bring a child into this world of control and abuse. What was I thinking? I did not know how I was going to tell Ron. I had very little communication with my parents, who I missed so much. Plus, if I was being honest with myself, if this abuse continued, I was not sure what may happen to both the baby and me. I was not raised in a religious home at all, but I believed there was a God. I remember someone telling me that if ever I needed something or was in trouble to call out to him. So, I did. I cried out, asking God why this happened and why I was continuously being beaten by someone who said he loved me. As I cried, I held my tummy. I was so lost at that moment and not sure which way to go. The craziest thing happened next. As I was asking God why, I felt movement in my tummy for the first time. It felt only like butterflies, but I felt it! "Thank you," I said. A peace came over my body; and I just knew everything was going to be okay.

I did not know my next step. But I knew I had to talk with my parents first. I remember coming to school that morning and asking the office if they could contact my parents for me. I needed them to come to the school. I had a cell phone, but Ron would take it away each morning I went to school, as he said I did not need it. You see, Ron drove me to and from school every day, so he always knew my exact whereabouts. So much control. I remember the principal asking if she could have the School Resource Officer join in with my parents, and I remember feeling a bit scared as I did not want to get in trouble. Now when I think about it, you were the best thing that happened. It's like you came into my life as my guardian angel. My parents came in that morning, and when I saw them, I ran into my mom's arms. I missed them so much and I was so sorry. Both my mom and dad held me as I sobbed into their shoulders, and as I calmed down, we made our way into the principal's office and sat down. They had been so worried about me. I remember you introducing yourself to me and my parents and telling us a bit about who you were. I knew right at that moment I was in good hands. I began to tell my parents about the beatings and about being pregnant. My mom put her arm around me and let me know it was going to be okay, they were here. I knew I needed to leave Ron but was not sure how I could make it happen. Now, being pregnant with his baby made things a lot more difficult. Constable S., I remember you looking into my eyes and I saw such compassion and empathy for me there, and I felt like I wasn't alone. The four of us began to put together a safety plan.

I knew I needed to tell Ron I was pregnant, but I was so afraid of what would happen, especially if I did it alone with him. So, we figured out a plan to meet him at a coffee shop with my parents. It was a neutral location and in public. I remember thinking about all the ways this could go wrong, but still felt at peace. Constable S., I knew that whatever the outcome, I was going to be okay. My parents arranged to meet me after school at the coffee shop, which was just beside the school. Once the plan was in place, they left the school, and I went to class. I asked one of my friends if I could borrow her cell phone to call Ron. I asked him to please meet me at the coffee shop after school. He agreed. The final bell rang at the end of the day. I stopped by the office to see if you were there. I saw you were with another student, so I waited. I remember feeling a sense of empowerment come over me, like I was going to be okay no matter what happened. You popped your head out of the principal's office and said hi. I think I just wanted to know that you were there and that you knew I was heading out. I remember you hugged me and told me, "You got this!" I made my way out of the school and over to the coffee shop. I saw that my parents were already there along with Ron. They had met one time before, so it wasn't as awkward as it would have been if this was the first time they met. I found a table and everyone sat down. Ron did not look happy, but that was okay, as he never seemed to be. I thanked everyone for coming, and then I looked at Ron and told him I was pregnant. His face turned white, and he asked how this happened as we only had sex one time. I said to him that all it took was ONE TIME! Well, he stood up and told me that I was not going to keep it and that I had to have an abortion. My parents stayed very calm and held my hand, and as they did, I felt a peace come over me. I let Ron know that I was not going to have an abortion as I did not agree with that and that I would have the baby. I would then decide if I would keep the baby or put it up for adoption. Well, he would not have it and he hit the table hard, knocking over his drink and spilling my parents' coffee. He looked at me and with rage in his eyes, yelled "You bitch. Why are you trying to ruin my life? I hate you and we are done. I will make sure you do not have this baby." He marched out of the coffee shop, slamming the door. Well, I thought, I know what his answer was. My parents looked at me and shook their heads. They knew this was going to be a battle, but they knew that if we stood together, we could get through this. I remember calling you and letting you know what had happened.

At that moment, Candace took a long pause. I could tell that she was replaying the memory in her head. I remembered that day very clearly, as I had indeed received a call from Candace after the coffee shop incident.

I had been waiting to see how the meeting went. I had a chance to investigate who Ron was. He had been charged numerous times with domestic assault as well as stalking. His motto seemed to be, "If I can't have her, no one can." I was concerned not only for Candace's safety, but also her baby's. I had learned over my past years in policing that these situations can change in a second and the outcome is often not good. I asked her where she was at that moment, and she said she was heading home with her parents. I told her to wait there, as I wanted to come and have a chat with them. I walked over to the coffee shop, and as I walked past a black Honda Civic, I noticed Ron sitting in the passenger's seat, talking to another male. He looked up as I stopped at the car. I smiled and motioned him to roll down his window. He was polite as he greeted me. I asked both boys what they were doing, and I was told they were waiting for someone. I asked who and Ron said, "Candace." I told him they should just leave, as I was going to be meeting with her and was not sure how long the meeting would last. He shook his head, said "whatever," and drove off. As he did, I made note of the license plate. I watched as the car turned the corner to make sure he had left the area. I made my way inside the coffee shop and met up with Candace and her parents. I hugged Candace and felt her melt into my arms. Then the tears started. "Constable S. I was so scared but did not want Ron to see my fear. I was not expecting him to react the way he did. I knew he would not be happy, but what he said really threw me off. To be honest, I believed his words and they scared me."

I had Candace and her parents sit down, and we began to set out a safety plan. For starters, one of her parents would drive her to and from school each day and I or the principal would walk her out. To some, this may have sounded a bit overboard. However, I had dealt with cases like this when I worked in the Domestic Conflict Unit. You never knew what the abuser was thinking or what their next move may be. Safety was the number one priority. I let Candace know that at any time she felt unsafe or had an uneasy feeling to let someone know. I also let her and her parents know about Ron's history of abuse and that I feared he meant what he said. Candace's dad said they had an alarm system at home and would make sure it was always on. I asked them if they needed anything else from me at that moment, and they said that they did not. I walked them out of the coffee shop, looked around to see if the Honda Civic had come back, and saw that the coast was clear. As we arrived at their car, Candace's mom turned around to hug me and as she did, whispered, "Thank you for bringing our daughter back to us." I told her that I would hope for the same if I were in this situation. She smiled at me. Candace came over, gave me a hug, and said, "See you in the morning." I could tell she felt more at ease. I waved goodbye and headed back to the school. Once inside, I notified my supervisor about what had happened and the plan that had been put in place. I wanted to make sure he was up to date just in case anything happened. Just another day in high school.

Over the next few weeks, I would see Candace arriving at school smiling and glowing. I would wave to her mom as she drove away. Then one day, as Candace and I were walking out of the front doors of the school, I noticed that same black Honda Civic waiting across the street from the campus. I stopped Candace and asked her to go back inside. I looked over to see who was in the vehicle. I noticed Ron in the driver's seat. I could not visibly see anyone else, but that did not mean there was only one person. I slowly made my way up to the car, and as I approached it, Ron rolled down the window. Ron said, "Hello Constable. How are you today?" I said that I was good and asked him what he was doing out there. He told me he was just hanging. I informed him that if he was not waiting for anyone that he was to leave the area, as he was not welcome there. Ron gave me the middle finger and drove off, squealing his tires as he did. I went back inside the school and asked Candace to see if her mom would come inside the school once she arrived. I was thinking that it may be time to look into securing a restraining order. It seemed that Ron was not getting the message, and my gut was telling me he really did not want to. Once Candace and her mom came into the office, I spoke to them regarding the process to obtain a restraining order and strongly urged them to explore it more. I walked with them out of the school and had a quick look around. No black Honda. They got into their car and drove away. I received a call from Candace and her mom that evening to let me know that she was being placed on bed rest. The stress was causing her blood pressure to rise extremely high, and her doctor felt for this last bit of her pregnancy, she needed to take care of herself and the baby. I let her know I was here if she needed anything and to keep me posted. I would try to stop by and check in on her in a week. After I hung up the phone, something in my gut was telling me to check in on her in a couple of days instead of a week. I felt that something was brewing, but I was not sure what.

The next few days were uneventful. There was no sign of Ron and things were pretty drama-free which for high school was amazing. I kept thinking about Candace and what she had gone through. That girl had shown such strength, and I was so proud of her. It had been just over a week since I had last checked in, so I gave her mom a call. I was informed that Candace had been taken into the hospital that morning as her baby was ready to enter the world. I was so excited. Her mom said she would let me know when I could come and visit Candace, as that was one thing she had asked me to do earlier on, to come and meet her daughter. I told her mom to keep me posted. About an hour later, I received a text message from Candace with a picture of baby Emily. It brought back such beautiful memories of when my son was born and the joy that it brought me. I could feel that through the picture. I texted her back that I would come and visit her the next day. I went home that night with such a peace in my heart. The next morning, I headed to the police district office and changed into my uniform. I signed out a police car and texted Candace to see if she was awake. There was no response. I thought I would head to the hospital anyway. A call came over the radio regarding an unwanted guest at the hospital, right where I was headed. I tried calling Candace but there was still no answer. My mind started wondering if this call had something to do with her ex-boyfriend, Ron. I asked dispatch if they had the name of the unwanted guest. My instinct was correct. Ron was trying to get into the hospital to see her. I guess he had been stopped once he got to the maternity floor. He had begun to argue with the nurses and security was called. He then began to fight with security, so then the police were called in. I let dispatch know I was heading that way and that I knew who this kid was and why he was there. I asked for backup, as I did not know what may come of this call. I turned on my lights and sirens and made my way through traffic. Sometimes I had to shake my head and wonder how some people were able to get their driver's licenses, because I had seen so many different types of driving when drivers see or hear lights and sirens. Now, I would expect that the cars would pull to the side and traffic would part like the Red Sea, but that never happens. I had one driver stop right in front of me, another pulled to the left and then realized they should have pulled to the right so crossed over right in front of my pathway to go to the right side. Oh my goodness, people! I was surprised that there were not more accidents with bad drivers and police cars. Just saying! I finally pulled into the front of the hospital, let dispatch know I was there, and headed up to the maternity ward. I ran out of the elevator and saw security trying to control Ron. By this time, Ron was so angry that he was using all parts of his body to fight, including his teeth. As I ran towards the three of them, I called out to Ron. For a moment he stopped fighting and looked over to me. That was just enough time for security to take him down to the ground and restrain him. As he was on the ground, I knelt beside him and quietly spoke to him. "Ron, what happened here today? Why were you fighting security and what were you doing here? You know you were not supposed to come here or be around Candace. What happened?" Security handcuffed Ron and turned him over so he could sit up. He looked at me with so much anger in his eyes. "This is my baby, and I am going to take it from Candace. She was not supposed to have that baby in the first place, and she does not deserve it now." I knew Ron was angry, but I did not realize that his rage had continued and that it was now to this point.

The backup police unit had arrived and would deal with Ron out front for the time being. I made my way to the nurses' station and asked what room Candace was in. As I entered the room, I saw a young, terrified girl lying in a hospital bed unable to make sudden moves. She looked up at me and started to cry. She had heard all the commotion outside and heard Ron screaming her name and how he wanted to take the baby. Luckily, her parents had been there and had held her. She was still a child and needed the comfort of her parents' arms. I let her know she was safe, and that Ron was in custody. I told her that I was just going to talk to the nurse quickly and then I would be back. I headed to the nurses' station and asked to speak with the head nurse. She knew a bit about what had occurred, and I gave her a rundown of what the history was between Ron and Candace. I asked if we could get Child and Family Services to give me a call, and I also contacted our Domestic Conflict Unit to update them and get them involved. I had a strong suspicion that this was not over.

I headed back to see Candace and her parents and updated them on the actions I had taken and who I had contacted. As of that moment, I knew that Ron had been charged with assaulting a peace officer and resisting arrest. He was being held for now. I was not holding my breath that he would be held for long, but I did not let Candace or her parents know that. The nurse came into the room and let me know that they would be releasing Candace and baby Emily in two days. That gave me a couple of days to figure out a safety plan with the Domestic Conflict Unit, if one would be needed. Once the situation had calmed down, I was able to spend some time with Candace and I got to hold and cuddle baby Emily. Oh, how I love the smell of a new baby and the warmth and joy they bring. I said my goodbyes and headed out to my car. The day was not even half over and so much had already happened. As I drove to the high school, Ron's words continued to play back in my head. This was someone who would not stop until they had control, and I was not sure what he was capable of, if I was being honest. Once I arrived at the school and sat down in my office, I sent an email to Candace's mom regarding the restraining order and if they had looked into it. I wanted to make sure they had all the needed information to make a decision. The message came back that they had indeed looked into it and had applied for one. Now it was a waiting game. I knew that if Ron remained in custody, Candace and her family would be safe. Candace returned home two days later and was feeling good. She texted me that she missed her friends at school and that having a brand-new baby was a lot of work. She was so right. It was not an easy task, but such a rewarding one. I let her know that she was in my prayers. I continued to check in with Candace on a weekly basis, and she continued to send me pictures of Emily and marvel at how fast she was growing. It had been three months and Ron remained in custody. This was good news, as Candace could begin back to her schooling with the help of her parents to look after Emily. A few more months went by. I then got news that I would be moving to another school, as I was needed to help put out some fires. I let Candace know that I was leaving but that I was only a phone call away.

I had moved schools and several months had gone by. I had lost touch with Candace and had heard nothing further about Ron. I spent four months at this new school, and then summer hit, and school was out. Life got busy, and when August rolled around, I was informed that I had been asked back to the school where Candace was attending. I had not spoken with her for several months at that point and assumed all was going well, and baby Emily was probably growing like a weed. It was a crisp morning at the beginning of September and little did I know that Candace would soon come back into my life.

As I had mentioned at the beginning of the chapter, I had just pulled up to the high school and saw Candace, noticing that she had recently been crying. She came into my office, gave me a big hug, and said she was so glad I was back. Emily was just about eight months old at that point. I could not believe how fast the time had gone by. I asked her what was going on that had made her so upset. She began her story:

> For the past few months, everything was quiet. I had applied for a restraining order, but because Ron was still in custody, the judge felt it was not needed. Emily has brought so much joy to our family and has continued to grow and change. Two days ago, I received a text from a number I did not recognize. It said, 'Bitch, your days are numbered. Enjoy the last days with the baby as she will not be yours much longer.' I was sick to my stomach as I knew exactly who that text was from, but I could not prove it. I am constantly looking over my shoulder and watching everyone around me. If it was Ron, I am not sure what he is capable of, but I have my suspicions. Can you please check to see if Ron is out of jail and if so, what can I do to protect myself? What rights does Ron have?

As I sat back in my chair, I could feel her pain. This was supposed to be a beautiful time with her daughter. Instead, she was living in fear. I made a few phone calls and found out that Ron had been released. I had a contact in Family Law and gave him a call to find out what rights both Candace and Ron each had. I had Candace speak to the lawyer. While she was speaking to him, I began to put together a safety plan for Candace and Emily. It was time to head back to the courts to apply for the restraining order. I knew it would not solve everything, but it was a start. Candace hung up the phone and I could tell by the look on her face that the news she received was not what she had been hoping to hear. Ron still had rights, even though there were threats happening; however, there were ways to work around this. I gave Candace a hug and we headed to the police car. As we drove down to the courthouse, Candace sat quietly in the passenger seat. I could tell her mind was spinning in so many directions. I asked if she wanted to talk or just listen to some music. She asked for the music, so Top 40 it was. We arrived at the courthouse. Candace and I went inside and made our way to where we would apply for the order. Candace spoke with the desk clerk, filled out all the information that was needed, and was told to sit and wait. Ten minutes later, both Candace and I were asked to go into the judge's chambers, as she wanted to speak with us about the application. We walked in, said hello to the judge, and took a seat. I had dealt with many judges over my career in law enforcement, but I could tell that Candace was both anxious and nervous. I leaned over and took her hand. As I did, she squeezed my hand so hard. I let out a light laugh, and the judge asked if everything was okay. I informed her that this was Candace's first time in a judge's chambers and that she was nervous. What I saw next warmed my heart. The judge came out from behind her desk, pulled up a chair next to Candace, and sat down. She then had a beautiful conversation with Candace about what was going on, how Candace was feeling regarding Ron being around, and what her fears were. Candace was fully transparent and honest, and I could tell that the judge respected that. The judge turned to me and said, "This is a very bright and well-spoken young lady you have here. I am saddened that she is going through all this at such a young age. I am granting the restraining order and I hope this all gets sorted out for the good of both Candace and her daughter. No mother ever wants to see her daughter have to deal with this." I thanked the judge, and as I looked over at Candace, tears were streaming down her face. She gave the judge a hug, looked at me, and gave me a hug too. As we were leaving the chambers, Candace looked at the judge and said, "Thank you for believing me," before we headed out of her office. Once outside the courthouse, I asked Candace how she was feeling. She said good but knew this was only the beginning. She knew Ron had a history of domestic assaults and no matter what, she wanted to make sure her family was safe. I contacted the Domestic Conflict Unit (DCU) and had Candace speak to one of the detectives. Now that a restraining order was in place, that gave the police more to work with. As soon as I dropped Candace off back at the school, I was going to meet up with another officer so they could serve Ron with the order. I knew it was just a matter of time before we would hear from Ron again. We made it to the school, and as Candace opened the car door, she looked over and said thank you. I headed off to meet the other officer, who I had asked to do some checkups on Ron and where he may be. He was not hard to locate, which was good. I met with the officer, handed over the restraining order, and he went and served the order to Ron. I was informed that Ron ripped the order up right in front of the officer and told him to F off. Well, this was going to be fun.

I contacted the DCU detective and let them know what had happened. They let me know that they would make sure to begin to look closely at this file and at Ron. These types of offenders can be more dangerous, as you never know what they will do next. I let Candace and her parents know that the order had been served. I also asked them to document everything that seemed a bit out of the ordinary, including if they noticed different cars driving up and down their street at certain times. They said they would keep a close eye out. I also ensured that Candace's parents would pick her up and drop her off like before, just as a precaution. All three were happy that things were in place, and they continued to live life as they had been. They did not want to live in fear. Over the next few weeks, all was going well. Fall was in full swing, and you could even feel a bit of a colder nip in the air. I would see Candace in the halls, happy and just being the joyful person that she was. Little did we know that all was about to change.

Candace was home alone with Emily while her parents had gone out for dinner. She was sitting and watching a show when her phone buzzed. She looked at the text message and it said you will never be safe. She did not recognize the number. She texted her mom to let her know about the text. Suddenly, there was a knock on the door. The knocks turned to banging, and someone yelled to open the door. Candace was scared and dialed 911. While talking to the 911 dispatcher, she noticed people trying to look through the window, so she hid. The banging on the door continued and the dispatcher said she could hear it. She ran upstairs and grabbed Emily, who was sound asleep, and took her into her parents' room, where she locked the bedroom door. Then she made her way into the ensuite and locked that door, as well. The dispatcher let her know that the police were on the way and told her to try to stay calm. That evening, I was home and relaxing when I received a call from our police dispatch. She informed me what was going on at Candace's residence and that police were on their way. I let her know that I feared the worst and that if this was Ron, he would not stop until he had killed her. I grabbed my keys and drove as fast as I could to the district office to get changed. It felt like I was moving at lightning speed as I changed into my uniform, signed out a car, and with lights and sirens going, made my way to the scene. I contacted the street sergeant to let him know that I was on my way and to give him the background on this call. Once he was aware, he went over the radio to ask anyone who could get there quickly to head that way. All units possible. I texted Candace to see what was happening and she said she was on with 911, but she could still hear the pounding on the door, and it sounded like they would break down the door. Just as she said that dispatch informed us that the intruders had gotten inside the house. It was now a race against time to get there. I heard over the radio that a unit had arrived. I pulled up and noticed the black Honda Civic on the side of the street across from the residence. I radioed in the license plate. Guess what? It came back as being owned by Ron. Over the air, I let the officers know there was a restraining order in place, and it contained the clause that police could use whatever force necessary.

I texted Candace that the police were there. The responding units headed inside the house, calling out as they did. There were two offenders who were taken into custody outside the front window. They had been trying to hide in the bushes. As the officers entered the house, they could hear pounding coming from a door upstairs. As they made their way up the stairs, they could see the master bedroom door had been broken and there were two males trying to get through the ensuite door. The officers yelled for the two offenders to get their hands up. As I made my way up the stairs, I could hear both Candace and Emily crying through the ensuite door. My heart was beating so fast. As I turned towards the master bedroom, I saw that one of the offenders was Ron. I let the officers know who he was and that the restraining order was against him. Both males were taken away in handcuffs. I ran to the ensuite door and let Candace know it was me. She unlocked the door and swung it open. She flew into my arms sobbing. As I held her, I saw that baby Emily was lying on the bathroom floor in a blanket crying as well. Holding onto Candace in one arm, I went and picked up Emily in the other and the three of us hugged. I told Candace that she had done so good, and I was so proud of her. As I led Candace out of the ensuite and bedroom and down the stairs, her parents ran in through the open front door. They hugged her so tightly and all three cried. I was still holding onto Emily, staring at this innocent child, knowing how close she had come to her life being forever changed that night. God had his angels surrounding these two. He had a purpose for their lives, and I was excited to see what was to come. Candace took Emily and hugged her. I gave the four of them some time, and I went outside to see who else had been arrested. Ron sat in the back of a police car with a smirk on his face. Three of his friends were chatting with different officers. One of the officers came over to update me on what they had found out. First off, Ron had a large knife on him as well as a bat and rope in the trunk of his car. The three other boys were just along for the ride. They all thought Ron just wanted to scare Candace. They had not realized his intentions and knew nothing about the restraining order. I went back inside and let Candace and her parents know what was going on and that all was good. Candace was now safe. Police helped Candace's dad fix the door the best they could until it could be looked at the next day. I asked the family if they wanted to go someplace else for the night, and they said they felt better being at home. I gave them all hugs, let Candace know I would contact her in the morning, and said goodbye. I thanked the other officers for all their help and asked if they needed anything else. I would put my statement on the report when I returned to the district office. My day was finally over.

Candace was very fortunate to have parents who supported her throughout her journey, as well, and had found someone to trust and talk with and provide a safe place for her. Not all youth have this available to them, and sometimes they have no place to turn. Both eating disorders and domestic abuse are happening in every walk of life, every class system, and every culture. I think sometimes we forget that this can happen to our own youth, or youth we know and interact with every day. It does not always look the same, and the effects may not always be the same. As the adults in these youths' lives it is so important to make sure to look out for the small things: the skipping meals, the change in behavior, the clothing styles, or with friendships. Each of these shifts in behaviors is worth an important conversation that can save a life.

CHAPTER 7

Finding Light in the Darkness: A Reflection on Suicide and the Search for Meaning

Jackie's Story

How many of us as parents know someone or have even struggled ourselves with suicidal tendencies? It is not an easy topic to have a conversation about, especially when it involves our own kids or kids we know. What if we were able to have that crucial conversation? Could that save a life, or give hope to someone who felt that there was no hope left?

The day started like any other day. Driving to the district office at 5:00 a.m. to get into my uniform before heading off to the high school, I knew today would be busy since the grade twelve graduation was just around the corner, and the buzz was in the air. Grade twelve pranks were being whispered about in the halls, and I could just imagine what this year may bring. Last year, some kids had released crickets in the vents and let off stink bombs in the washrooms, and of course we had our variety of streakers that made their way through the school. Never a dull moment in the halls of a high school. Oh, how I loved my job. As I was retrieving the keys to my police vehicle, I received a text from the school Principal, Mr. Jones. One of the parents of a student had received comments from some of their daughters' friends. These comments were regarding Facebook messages sent from their daughter last evening. As soon as I got into the vehicle, I called the principal for more information. The student's name was Jackie, and her parents wanted to speak with me.

Jackie was an honor student, was loved by her teachers and fellow students, and was a beautiful young lady. She was athletic, with blond hair and blue eyes, and as others would say she was perfect. She had her pick of any university, as they all seemed to want her, and she was never short of friends as everyone wanted to be seen with her. I had met her during one of the school pep rallies because she was also part of student council. She came across as happy and having it all together. So, what were these messages all about? I contacted Jackie's parents as soon as I got off the phone with Mr. Jones. Jackie's mom, Beth, answered and placed me on speaker phone since her dad, Al, was there as well. I introduced myself and asked how I could help. I could feel the eeriness in the room as it came through the phone. Like there was more to the story, but neither of her parents wanted to be the one to talk first. I first let them know that I was on my way over to their house and then I asked about the Facebook messages. Beth piped up, and through her tears began to explain what was going on:

> Last night, Jackie came home as usual, went up to her room, and instead of coming down to chat, she stayed upstairs with her door closed. This was not like her, so I knocked on her door. She asked what I wanted, and I asked her if we could chat for a few minutes. She opened

the door, which had been locked (Jackie never locks her door), and I could tell she had been crying. I asked her if she was okay. She said she was fine but then broke down sobbing. I had not seen my little girl cry like this since her first breakup. It had been a while. Jackie looked at me and said she had just been informed that she had not gotten into the university program or university that she wanted to go to. She could not understand why, as her marks were high and everything else that she sent in was done to the best that she could. What did she miss? I explained to her that maybe there were a lot of top applicants this year and that they had too many choices and not enough openings. She did not like that answer. Jackie then let me know that she had had a fight with her best friend that afternoon and they would not be attending the graduation banquet together. Now that was surprising, as these two had been best friends for fifteen years. I asked Jackie if she wanted to tell me more about the fight. She explained that her best friend had heard from someone that Jackie and her best friend's boyfriend had been seen talking in the hall during class change, and supposedly Jackie had been laughing and touched his arm. At that moment I was trying to get my head around what she had just told me when I noticed a message appear on her computer. It was from her best friend, and it said that she hoped Jackie would die in her sleep as no one deserved Jackie's friendship.

I could not believe it had gotten this bad so fast. I went over to Jackie and held her in my arms as she just sobbed into my shoulder. I asked her if there was anything that her dad or I could do then, and she said she was hungry. I went downstairs and put some lasagna on a plate for her and took it back up to her room. Jackie said she was just going to eat and watch a bit of TV. I asked her that if she did shut her door if she would please not lock it, and she said she would keep it unlocked. I then asked her the toughest question I have had to ask her in a long time; I asked her if she felt like hurting herself. She told me I did not have to worry. Constable, something in my gut said that was not the truth.

As I listened to Beth tell her story, I could sense a bit of urgency in her voice. So, I asked her what had happened next. Beth continued her story:

I knocked on Jackie's door about an hour later and there was no answer. My heart started pounding. Should I have listened to my gut? I opened the door, yelling her name, and as I opened the door, I saw she had fallen asleep. I was so scared of what I was going to find on the other side of that door. I took a couple of deep breaths to calm my heart down. I turned off her TV, took her half-eaten plate of lasagna, covered her up, and left the room. I made sure to leave her door open just a crack, enough that if there were movement, I would know. I made my way down to the kitchen and told Al about what had just happened. I told him that something in my gut was not at peace, and I was not sure what it was. He said we would check on her before we went to bed and then chat more with her in the morning. Around 11:00 p.m., when I went upstairs to get ready for bed, I saw that her door was closed and the light was on in her room. I knocked on her door and she opened it. Jackie had gotten into her pajamas and thanked me for covering her up and turning off her TV. She said it was quite an emotional day and that she must have dosed off from exhaustion. She said she was feeling a bit better and was going to head to bed.

What I did not realize was she had been on her computer sending out farewell messages on Facebook. Al and I went to sleep, and at around 5:00 a.m. my phone started dinging with messages. It woke me out of a deep sleep. As I grabbed the phone to see what was going on, my heart sank. Parents of Jackie's friends were trying to contact me, as their kids had been receiving these Facebook messages from Jackie the night before. I jumped out of bed, turned on the light, and ran to Jackie's room. Her door was again closed and again locked. I pounded on the door screaming her name and Al ran towards the door and shouldered it to try and open it. The door broke open but there was no Jackie. I searched her room, every inch of it, and she was not there. Her computer was still on her desk, but her phone was gone. She left the car that she usually drives at home, as well. I have tried calling her phone but there is no answer. It does ring but no one picks up. Constable, I am unsure what to do next, but I am thinking the worst right now.

I let both Beth and Al know that I was almost to their house and as soon as I got there, we would figure out a plan. I hung up with Beth and called my supervisor to get him up to speed on what I may be dealing with. I arrived at the residence and let my supervisor know that I would keep him posted as I continued to find out more information. I got out of the car and before I went up to the front door, I had a quick look around the outside of the house. I did not see anything that looked out of place, so I knocked on the door. Beth opened the door and ushered me inside as Al stood near the door. I introduced myself. I asked if I could have a look at her laptop and the Facebook posts that her friends were receiving. As Beth went upstairs to grab the computer, I asked Al if I could have a look around the house. I wanted to make sure that no area was left unsearched. As I looked around the house, I noticed beautiful pictures of Jackie and her parents everywhere. What was going through this young lady's head to disappear like this? I checked the whole residence and made my way back to the kitchen, where Beth had now returned with the laptop. Beth showed me the Facebook posts and I could understand why Jackie's friends were concerned. The posts read as if Jackie was saying goodbye for good. I knew I had to figure out a plan of action and fast. I excused myself and stepped outside to update my supervisor. I let him know what the posts read and informed him I would be heading to the school shortly to meet with the principal. I went back inside the residence and had Beth call Jackie's phone one more time. Again, it rang and then went to voicemail, which meant it was still on. I radioed dispatch and asked if they could ping this cell phone number. At least this would be a start in finding a possible location. By this time, a few friends had begun to arrive at Jackie's home, worried about her. I spoke to them, and the same words were repeated over again, "This is not like her at all."

I let Beth and Al know that I would keep them in the loop if I heard anything and vice versa and headed back to the school.

As I sat in the car, I began to prepare myself for several possible outcomes, as I did not know what I may be walking into. I had so many different emotions running through my body, I did not know what to feel at that moment. As I began to drive, dispatch came over the radio to let me know that Jackie's cell phone had been pinged near the area of the school. That was perfect, as I was already on my way there. As I pulled up to the school, I said a little prayer that God would prepare me for whatever was to come. I needed his strength, wisdom, and courage before I headed into the school. Once inside, I met with Mr. Jones. I let him know that Jackie's phone had been pinged somewhere around the area of the school. It was still a big area, but at least we had a tighter location. Several school staff, as well as other police officers, had gathered in the office and were wanting to help out. I needed the school thoroughly searched, as no one knew if Jackie had shown up here early that morning. Each person was given my cell number to let me know what area had been searched and whether anyone was located. Time was not on our side, as I did not know if this cry for help was now a race for time. As the staff and other officers began their searches, Mr. Jones and I began our own search. I remembered there was an area in the girl's locker room that was a bit more hidden and out of the way and decided to go check there first. Something in my gut told me to check there first. I had hoped that by reading the posts Jackie had made, something would jump out to me regarding a location or special place, but nothing was indicated. As I came upon the locker room door, I prayed as I walked through the door frame for strength and courage. I called out, "Is anyone in here? Jackie, are you in here? It's Constable Sheremata." I could not hear anything, so I made my way to the back area. As I turned the corner, I stopped in my tracks as I could see someone lying against the inside of one of the bathroom stalls. The stall door was closed and as I looked up, I saw a rope hanging from the pipes in the ceiling. I felt my heart skip a beat. I ran over to the next open stall and hopped onto the toilet seat to see over the top of the closed-door stall. There was Jackie, sitting on the ground with the rope ready to go around her neck. I yelled to Mr. Jones that I found her and as she heard my voice, she looked up at me and said, "I couldn't do it. I am so sorry for all this trouble I caused." I asked her if she could unlock the door for me and she did. I slowly opened the door and had a brief but good look around to make sure I noted every detail of what I saw. I went inside the stall and asked her if I could sit with her. Jackie remained on the floor while I sat on the toilet seat. I asked her if it was okay that I let the others know she had been located, and she gave me a nod. I radioed dispatch and the other officers listening that she had been located and alive. I asked for the Emergency Medical Services (EMS) to make there way to my location to check Jackie out. I also asked dispatch to have her parents contacted that she had been located and was safe. As I sat with Jackie, a memory came over me of a time when I was in her shoes, feeling that hope was gone and that life would be so much easier if I was not around anymore. Tears filled my eyes as I looked at her, grabbed onto her hand and let her know that she was very loved, and that the world IS a better place because she is in it. Jackie could not hold it in any longer and all the pain and adrenaline came out of her in sobs. As the tears continued down my cheeks, I leaned over to her and just held onto her. She was safe.

The medics placed Jackie on a stretcher and began to look her over. As they did, I looked again in the stall to see what exactly could have been the result. The rope had been tied to the pipe and all she had to do was place it around her neck. I had no words. As the medics began to wheel her out, Jackie called out to me. I went over to her, and she asked if I would ride with her to the hospital. I told her I would. I just had to talk with the other officers and let her parents know which hospital she would be taken to. As we got to the front foyer of the school, the staff and officers who had helped with the search were gathered, and as Jackie was wheeled past them, I looked and noticed that not a dry eye was among them; even the officers. Later, I asked the staff involved what they were thinking at that time, and each of them, including the officers, said that it made them realize that this could have been their kid. It hit many close to home. Once Jackie was inside the ambulance and her parents had a chance to speak with her, Beth made her way over to me. She opened her arms and gave me the biggest bear hug ever. As she did, I felt her body release the weight of the world and she quietly let her tears flow. She whispered to me, "I cannot thank you enough. You have such an amazing way with these youth. They trust you and know you have no judgment towards them. That is such a gift." I thanked her for her kind words, jumped into the ambulance with Jackie, and headed to the hospital. Every day was a new adventure and every day, I had the opportunity to have an impact in these youths' and parents' lives. What a true blessing.

We never know what a person may be feeling. Just taking the time to say "hi" to someone or smiling at them can be the difference between life and death. That person we walked by and said good morning to, or that person we paid it forward to in the coffee line, they may have been contemplating taking their life that day because they felt unseen. You may have just showed them that they matter and are seen, and that is a huge light in the darkness.

Be kind, as you never know what someone has been or is going through.

CHAPTER 8

Why Won't This Pain Stop: Looking Beyond the Surface of Self-Harm

Emily's Story

It's often said that we never truly know the battles others are fighting. Behind every smile or seemingly ordinary moment, there can be a world of pain that can be hidden. It is a reminder that beneath the surface, many are enduring silent storms, and we need to approach each other with kindness and compassion.

I had noticed Emily around the high school. She was a beautiful young lady who seemed to keep to herself. I had seen her on several occasions hanging out with a group of girls. When she was with them, she always smiled and seemed happy. Little did I know that this young girl was suffering so much each day that in order to alleviate her pain, she would hurt herself.

I was in my office at the high school and received a call from one of the teachers. He asked if he could come and have a quick chat with me, that it was regarding one of his students. I told him to come by as I would be here. A few minutes later there was a knock on my office door and Mr. Evans stuck his head in. He came in and closed the door. I could tell by the look on his face that this was something serious. "Thank you so much for seeing me. I have this young lady named Emily in my class and over the last few weeks, I have noticed her behavior changing. She has begun to withdraw more, and she has gone from a sort of smiley person to a sad person. I have also noticed when she bends down to pick things up, like her bag or a book, she winces in pain and holds her stomach. This last time I noticed I asked if she was okay. She said she was, and that was the end of the conversation. You know when you have that feeling that something is just not right? Well, that is the feeling I have but I cannot pinpoint why I have that feeling. I thought maybe you could check in with her." I told him I would check in with Emily, and I thanked him for letting me know and caring so much for his students. He left my office and I headed to the main office to find out what class Emily had at that time. She had math. I called up to the math room and asked her teacher to let her know to come and see me at the break, as I did not want to make it public knowledge that I wanted to see her. The bell rang about twenty minutes later, and as I was finishing up a report, there was a knock on my office door. I got up and said to come in. Emily poked her head in and said she had been told to come see me. I welcomed her in and asked her to have a seat. As she did, I noticed she winced in pain and held her stomach, but she tried to hide it. I got up, introduced myself to her, and went to close the door. I did not want her to feel awkward, so I began to ask her how she was enjoying this school year and how her friends were. I sat down next to her and asked her how she was doing. "I'm okay. School is going well, and I am enjoying it." I then asked her if everything at home was okay. She shook her head, looked up at me, and tears began to well up in her eyes. Then the tears began to flow, and as they did, Emily told me her story:

Things are not okay at home. I come to school every day trying to force a smile on my face, but I am dying on the inside. My parents have had issues for a while and even went for counseling. The yelling and slamming doors were getting to be too much for me. My heart would ache each time I heard my mom crying. I would try and give her a hug but each time she would push me away. I have a younger brother and I began to see him start screaming when my parents would fight. Then Dad would yell at him to stop, and Mom would then yell at Dad to be quiet. It was a constant cycle that would not end.

Each time the yelling began, I would go into my room and try to listen to music. But over time that was not enough to soothe me. One of my friends had told me that when she was hurting inside, she would either cut or burn her inner thigh and the pain from that would get her mind off the hurt she was feeling. At first, I thought that sounded awful. But about two months ago, my heart hurt so much that I decided to try it. I used a razor and I cut two lines on my upper inner thigh. Wow, did it ever hurt, but I forgot what I was thinking about before, so it worked. There was not a lot of blood, which was good as I am not good with blood. I had a wet towel next to me, so I placed it on the cuts as they stung for a bit. "Hmm," I thought, that was not too bad, and my friend was right. I had forgotten about how sad I was feeling. I was feeling a bit lightheaded, so I drank some water. I got up, hid my razor in my sock drawer, put on my pajamas, and crawled into bed. The screaming had stopped, but there was an eerie silence that came over the house. I put on my headphones and drifted off to sleep. The next morning when I woke up, my inner thighs were quite tender. I crawled out of bed and took off my pajama pants. I noticed that the cuts were red, so I rubbed some polysporin on them, got into my clothes for school, and did my hair and makeup. I went downstairs and found my mom getting a bowl of cereal for my brother. I asked her how she was, and she said that she was fine. I grabbed a piece of toast and went to give my mom a hug, and she brushed me off yet again. I am not sure what I did but I was beginning to feel a bit rejected. I said goodbye and headed to school. Time to put on my smile and look happy. No one asked me if I was okay. I got home later that afternoon and like clockwork, the arguing began, along with the door slamming and swearing. I went back into my room, closed the door, and took out the razor. Cutting this time seemed so much easier. This continued for the next few weeks. It got to the point where the cutting was not enough, so I took a lighter and began to see how long I could hold a flame to the skin on my inner thigh until it really hurt. The first few times I could not hold it for long, but over time, I was able to hold it for a while; up to the point that my skin would bubble and blister. It hurt like hell, but I was able to drown out the screaming from my parents fighting.

Then one day, I came home after school, and the house was quiet. I called out to see if anyone was home. My dad came around the corner with a box in his hands. He said that he and mom were done, and he was moving out. I threw down my bag, screamed at the top of my lungs, and ran up into my room. I slammed the door and sobbed. What happened to this perfect family that I was supposed to have? What was going to happen to my brother and me? I grabbed my lighter, pulled down my jeans and began to hold the flame to the skin of my inner right thigh. That was it, I was now going to hold the flame there until my skin started to sizzle. I was so pissed off right then. The flame got so hot that I dropped the lighter. I looked at my thigh and man, I did some damage. Who cared? At least I was not feeling the pain inside my heart at that moment. I found some gauze and wrapped up my thigh. I hoped that it was not going to get infected.

Well, Dad moved out and it was now just my mom, my brother, and I. My mom became even more distant than before, and I had to take care of my brother. I would feed him and get him ready for bed at night and school in the morning. Mom would come downstairs, grab some food, and head back upstairs. This continued for several weeks. And guess what? I would show up at school every morning with a smile on my face and feeling like crap inside. When I would get home, I would knock on my mom's door to check in on her. This was not how I ever imagined life as a teen. I would get my brother into bed, say goodnight, and then head to my room and close the door. This one night, I was finding that neither the razor nor the burning was taking the pain away. I decided to try something else, I took the razor and cut open my stomach. This hurt something fierce.

*I wondered if there was something more drastic that I could
do to keep the outside pain stronger than my inside pain?
I found a way. Can I show you?*

Emily stood up from her chair, and as she did, she lifted her shirt
just above her tummy area and I gasped. The area was all infected,
and she had literally been carving out her stomach in a way that
was similar to the way we would carve out a pumpkin. Tears welled
up in my eyes as I could not hold them back. I had seen a lot in
my years as a police officer, but I had never seen anything like this.
This poor child was crying for help. I asked her if it would be okay
to take her to the children's hospital and have the injury assessed
by a doctor. She said yes. I also asked her if she had told her mom
anything about this and she said that she had not. I let her know
that I needed to contact her mom to let her know I was taking her
to the hospital, and all she said was, "Good luck with that." I was
not expecting that comment. I grabbed my keys and asked Emily if
she had everything she needed and she nodded. We walked out of
my office toward the main office. I stopped in, asked Emily to hang
on for a moment, and went to update the principal. As I informed
him, his face went white, as if he had seen a ghost. He sat down in
his chair and was speechless. I let him know I would update him.
Emily and I headed to my police car. I called my supervisor and let
him know what was going on and that I would keep him posted.
On the way to the hospital, Emily looked at me and asked what had
made me check in with her. I let her know that one of her teachers
had come down to say that he was worried about her. She smiled.
It was as if I saw a sense of relief come over her entire body. We
arrived and walked into the emergency. I knew that the staff would
be placing her in the mental health area, and I also knew that we

may be there for several hours before we were seen. They called Emily in, and she asked if I would come and sit with her while she waited. I said of course I would. I asked her if it was okay to contact her mom and see if she would come to the hospital. She smirked and said I could try. I stepped away from the area and called her mom. She answered the phone and I let her know where we were and what was happening. I asked her if she could come and be with her daughter while she waited. The answer was not what I was expecting. It was a hard no. Her mom said this was her trying to get attention, and she was not going to be a part of it. I could not believe what I was hearing. I thanked the mom for taking my call and hung up the phone. I was disgusted if I'm going to be honest. I made my way back to where Emily was waiting, and she knew from my face that the call had not gone well. "See, I told you. She is not coming, is she?" "Nope," I said.

We sat in silence for a few minutes. I was trying to process what had just happened. While we were waiting, Emily and I talked about life, her brother, the life that she had always hoped for, and what she wanted to be when she grew up. She was such a beautiful young lady both inside and out. As she talked, her face would light up with certain topics. Her brother was one of them. Five hours had passed and still no sign of seeing the doctor. I went to the nurse's desk and asked if they had any information on how much longer it would take until we were in the room. They could not tell me. I figured that would be the answer. One more hour passed, and Emily was finally called in. She walked into the room and gestured for me to come in with her. The doctor asked who I was and why I was with her. Well, I thought my uniform gave it away, but maybe not. Emily piped up, "This is my constable from the school who has been my only support. My mom won't be coming. I want the constable to stay here with me." You go girl! Way to take a stand. The doctor introduced himself along with the resident who was with him. He asked Emily why she was there and what he could do for her. She lifted her shirt over her tummy and showed him what she had shown me. The resident turned away in disgust. The doctor began to ask Emily questions about why she had done this and how she was feeling now. Emily also informed the doctor about her inner thigh and how that had made her feel. He asked if she could change into a hospital gown so he could have a better look. The doctor, resident, and I stepped out of the room so Emily could change into the gown. She opened the door, and we went back inside. She showed the resident and doctor her inner thigh. It was much worse than she had let on. It looked like she had second-degree burns, but I would wait to see what the doctor said. I was really hoping they would keep her in the hospital so she could start receiving the help that she needed. Her cry for help was so loud. The doctor wrote a prescription for a topical cream as well as some antibiotics for the infection that had started and told Emily she could get dressed. I was confused. Had he seen what I had seen and heard what I had heard? He, along with the resident and I, stepped out of the room. "I am confused doctor, as this child has been self-mutilating for a while, and it continues to get worse. This is such a huge cry for help. Is this not enough to keep her here and help her?" He looked at me and said, "If we kept every youth that cut or self-harmed, our beds would be full." My blood was boiling by this point. I could not hold my tongue anymore. "So, I guess she will have to be brought back in a body bag before you people do anything about it!" I was then informed that they would be submitting a formal complaint against me. All I could say was, "Good luck. Have at it."

Emily opened the door and walked out. She could tell by my face that something had just happened. I asked her if she was ready to go and she answered she was. We headed back to the car. Once she was seated inside, I stayed out and called my supervisor. I wanted to let him know a complaint may be coming my way from the doctor. He laughed and said he would be ready for it. I had been blessed with such an amazing supervisor. I got into the car, and we began to drive. I asked Emily if she wanted me to take her home. She said yes and then asked if I would come in and talk to her mom with her. I said I would for sure. I knew she needed all the support she could get. We arrived at her house and went to the front door. She opened it and we went inside. She called for her mom to come to the front so we could talk with her. Her mom came out, but I could tell by her facial expression that she was not happy about it. Emily told her mom what had been going on and then showed her mom her stomach area. Her mom fell to her knees and held onto Emilys hand. Her mom began to cry and through the tears told Emily she was so sorry. "I am so sorry for not listening to you and really seeing you. I am sorry that I continued to push you away. You did not deserve that. I am sorry that you have had to take all this on. I am sorry I have not been there for you." Her mom got up and hugged Emily. This was so beautiful to see. Her mom got it. I could tell Emily was very surprised at this response. This was not the mom that she had been living with for the past few years. But I also knew that this was the mom that Emily had yearned so much for. I said goodbye and left them to talk more about the day. I got back into the police car and drove back to the school. It had been a long day, but such a rewarding day. I had hoped that this story would have a happy ending, but I'm afraid it did not.

Emily and her mom had begun family counseling, and Emily was seeing a psychologist, as well. She had told her mom that she had stopped with self-harming. We would later find out that these feelings were way deeper than people had suspected. I had continued to check in with Emily. She said things were good, she had just gotten better at hiding things. Four weeks later, I received a frantic call from her mom that she could not get a hold of Emily and she was feeling very uneasy about it. I told her I would meet her at the house. Before I left, I checked to see if Emily had attended any of her classes that day. She had not. My stomach dropped. I was not feeling good about what we may be walking into. I headed to the car and got in. I began to drive to the residence and contacted dispatch with what information I knew. I asked if we could have Emergency Medical Service (EMS) standing by just in case, as well as another police unit. As I pulled up to the residence, my heart beat faster and faster. I hated these situations, as I could only think of the worst scenario as the outcome. I got out of the car and Emily's mom had just pulled up. I asked her if she wanted me to go on my own or if she wanted to come in with me. She said she wanted to come. I said a quick prayer for strength and courage and had Emily's mom unlock the front door. Both EMS and the other police unit had arrived, and I asked them to come in behind us. I walked in and called out to Emily. No answer. I asked the other unit to clear the main level and I was going to head upstairs with Mom and EMS. As I got to the top of the stairs, I noticed a closed door, and Emily's mom said that was Emily's bedroom. I knocked on the door, no answer. I opened the door while announcing I was coming in. There was Emily on her bed. She had not survived. I had so many emotions going through my body. I was so sad and felt hurt and pain for her mom. I was so angry at the doctor for not taking what Emily had told him to heart. Yet, at that moment, I felt a peace that Emily was not hurting anymore. Tears ran down my cheeks and I turned to Emily's mom and hugged her. No one should have to go through this, especially a parent. She looked at me and said, "Thank you for being there for Emily and supporting her when no one else was there for her. I feel like I failed her, and I will have to live with that for the rest of my life. I hope God can forgive me." I looked at her. "You have been forgiven. Now you need to forgive yourself."

We never know the silent struggles that people may be facing, and the pain people carry is often invisible. It's a reminder that empathy and understanding are crucial. Practicing empathy, offering support, encouraging professional help, and educating others to break the stigma are all so important. Your compassion and support can be the beacon of hope for those in need.

CHAPTER 9

Suffering in Silence:
The Silent Struggles of Bullying

Michelle's Story

Bullying is a pervasive issue that affects countless youth, often leaving lasting scars. The emotional, psychological and sometimes physical impact of bullying can shape a young person's life in profound ways. As caregivers, our role in recognizing, addressing and preventing bullying is crucial, and our empathy, vigilance, and proactive involvement can make a significant difference in a youth's life.

It was the start of a new year at the high school and the day of the big pep rally. The halls were full of students who were excited for the afternoon festivities. The football players were chanting as they made their way into the gym and the cheerleaders were getting ready for their performance. I stood by the gym doors as the students began to pour into the gymnasium, high-fiving the kids as they came by. I loved this time of year as it was so fresh and full of excitement and newness. Everyone, including the teachers, was excited to be back and in the swing of things. As I was preparing to welcome everyone back to school, I noticed a young girl out of the corner of my eye. I had not yet met her, but she stood out because she had very beautiful exotic features. As she looked in my direction, I caught her eye and noticed a sadness and hurt there. I gave her a smile. I was going to make sure I connected with her later that day. Something inside me said it was important to do.

The pep rally began, and the gym erupted in cheers. It was so amazing to see and feel the school spirit. Everywhere you looked, the smiles and laughter filled the room. Yet, when I came across the young girl I had noticed earlier, she was wiping away tears. Who was this girl and what was going on in her life? As the pep rally was winding down and students started heading back to class, I noticed this girl stayed seated on the bleachers. I walked over to where she was sitting and introduced myself. She told me her name was Michelle. I asked her if she was okay? She asked if she could come and talk with me in my office, and I told her that would work. I motioned to one of the teachers to let them know that I was heading out, and Michelle and I headed to my office.

As we were walking, I asked Michelle a few questions: what school she had come from, was she from here, and how she was finding high school. Michelle said she was from Calgary and came from the community middle school. She said she had been nervous about coming to grade ten, as the school was so much bigger than her middle school and she was afraid she may not fit in. As we made our way to my office, Michelle's phone started dinging with messages. It went six times in a row, and on the last time I noticed her face change. She had a look of pain and disgust. We walked into the office and I closed the door. As Michelle sat down, I looked at her and asked her what was going on. Michelle began her story:

Last year, there was this group of girls who were mean to all the other girls and guys in grade nine. They would try and find one thing about a person that was different or weird and then use it to torment them. At first, I had been part of this group until I began to see what they were doing and how it was hurting people. One of the boys in our class ended up committing suicide because of the things that this group was saying and spreading around about him. I was so devastated. You see, before the suicide, I had gone and spoken to the principal about what was going on and how far this bullying was being taken. I was informed that it would be investigated. The harassment continued and still nothing had been done. Someone must have found out that I had gone to the principal, because the next day, I was receiving messages all over social media about how this school would be better off without me here and how terrible it must be for my parents, having a loser like me as a kid. That evening, I sat down with my mom and dad and let them know about the messages. In all my years, I had never had something like this happen. While I was sitting with my parents, my phone continued to make a noise, informing me that there were messages and posts. I gave my phone to my mom, and as she and my dad scrolled through the posts and comments, tears welled up in her eyes. She could not understand how girls could be so mean and how others could continue to add fuel to the fire. The comments were everything from telling me to go kill myself to saying that no one liked me and that I was better off dead. Someone even commented on the method I should use to kill myself.

You know, no one knows how this begins to affect you unless they have experienced it themselves. I thought I was strong, and I had amazing support around me. But day after day as these messages and comments continued, each little stab began to hurt more and more. It was like being killed by a thousand stab wounds. My parents noticed my behavior change. I was missing school, staying in my room more, communicating less with them, and overall became very distant and closed off. My parents and I decided together that continuing to look at my phone was not doing me any good, so they asked me if they could keep it and monitor what was coming through. I agreed to it. My dad also felt it was time to contact the principal and have a meeting with him regarding the bullying. I agreed with that, as well. So, off the three of us went to the school and into a meeting with the principal. What a waste of time that was. The principal began his talk with kids will be kids and blah blah. I could not believe what I was hearing. I then spoke up and reminded him that I had already come to see him regarding this issue and how things were continuing and getting worse. He informed me that he did not have a magic wand. I was so angry. It felt like he was not wanting to deal with this. I know my parents were worried about me, but I was more worried about some of the other kids who had been targeted and did not have the strength or support that I had. I got up, opened the door, turned to the principal, and said this wasn't finished, and walked out the door and out of the main office. My parents followed. I could not believe that someone who was supposed to be in charge of youth and their livelihoods could be that dismissive. It was interesting because at that moment, I felt this sense of empowerment come over me. I felt I was able to deal with this and stand tall. I decided to head to class while my parents went home. I was not going to allow what the principal or these other kids said take me down. Remember that boy I had talked abut earlier, the one who had committed suicide? Well, his name was John. I knew him because we were both in art class together. He was a cool kid, very creative and so artistic. That day I had gone back to school I ran into him in the hall. We chatted for a moment, as the bell was about to ring, but we were going to touch base after class. I had seen his name come up numerous times as one of the kids being bullied and I wanted to find out how he was doing. As class ended, I overheard a few kids talking about John, and some of the comments that continued to be said about him. I asked one of the girls if they knew where it all started from, but everyone's lips were sealed. I wondered if it had been a friend of theirs, if they would have still kept their mouths shut. I was able to chat with John after class and we got talking about what had been circulating on social media. John told me how he was suffering in silence as no one knew the real pain that he was feeling. I told him that I completely understood. I asked him if he had talked to anyone about these feelings and he said that he hadn't. Looking back now, that was my first mistake. He needed an outlet and someone he could trust and felt safe with. I told him I was here for him and to please reach out. Well, the messages did not stop, and they continued to get meaner. I felt like I was part of that movie Mean Girls. I was trying so hard for this not to affect me, but it did. I could hear my mom's voice saying water off a duck's back . . . well this duck seemed to be a sponge and was soaking up way more than I should have been. My parents had mentioned that we should go to the police. I had thought about it, but I did not feel it was that big of a deal yet. Little did I know that not only would someone die, but this would follow me into grade ten.

Michelle looked up at me and I noticed her eyes glistening with tears. This young girl sitting in front of me was in so much pain yet trying to be strong. I handed her a Kleenex and she continued:

John passed away near the end of the school year, and I watched as that really took a toll on several kids. Grade nine graduation was so different. It was like there was this elephant in the room that no one wanted to talk about. I had heard that several parents had begun to come forward to the principal regarding these girls and the bullying. At least other kids were coming forward. Maybe that was the one positive that came out of John's death. Kids began to have voices and feel safe to come forward. I am not sure what the outcome was once the parents came forward. I had hoped the principal would start to realize this was a bigger issue and he needed to step in. I am thinking that was not the case because the bullying is still going on.

Michelle passed me her phone and I began to scroll through the comments and messages.I was floored by the things that were being said and the language that was being used by these youths. I asked her if I could do some digging into what had been done last year and told her that I would get back to her. She told me to also keep her phone, as it was doing nothing but making her upset. She texted her mom to let her know I would be keeping her phone for the time being. Her mom said that was a great idea. Michelle said thank you and headed to class. I had not been sitting there for more than three minutes and at least fifty comments and messages had come through. This was insane and out of control. I first contacted our principal to let her know what was going on and that I would be investigating this as it had started last year at the other school. I also let her know that I would be contacting the other principal, as I wanted to get his insight on what had happened and what had been done. I contacted the middle school and was informed that the principal was no longer there. He had been moved to a different school. So sad; instead of dealing with the injury, it got bandaged up and left to scar. I found out where he had gone and called that school. I was put through to his line and he picked up. As I began to tell him the nature of my call, he cleared his throat. I could sense a feeling of uneasiness coming through the phone. I asked him if he could explain to me his side of what had occurred and what action steps had been taken. I also informed him that the bullying was still happening by the same group of girls to the same youth as last year. He released a heavy sigh. I could tell that this was not something he was excited to talk about. He began to explain what happened:

> I had been hearing buzz around the school that there was a group of girls doing this, but no one had come forward at the time. Then Michelle came to see me and showed me her phone with the messages. To be honest, I could not believe these words were coming out of girls' mouths. They

were so vulgar and full of hate. I asked her if I could take a screenshot of the messages and she said yes. Once she left, I went into the assistant principal's office and let her know what was going on. Carlamay, last year was my first year as principal and it was so overwhelming and such a huge learning curve that I felt like I was underwater most of the year. So, when this issue came up, I thought I knew how to handle it, but it seemed to get worse before I could even get a grasp on it. Then, when the suicide happened and more parents began to come forward, I knew I was in trouble.

I let him finish and then I asked him why he did not ask for help from the School Resource Officer who had been at his school or even contacting the school district psychologist for some guidance. I was taken aback by the lack of knowledge and leadership skills that he had shown. He oversaw lives, and to feel so overwhelmed and not sure where to go for help raised several concerns for me. He said he was sorry that he had not dealt with the issue last year properly and that it had continued. I thanked him for his honesty, and I told him that I hoped he knew he could reach out for support, since we all need it no matter what area we work in. He was very grateful. I hung up the phone and began to look at all the messages that were coming through on Michelle's phone. I wanted to get a better understanding of who all was involved, both bullies and victims. It seemed there were four girls who were the key players and five (plus Michelle) potential victims. I wanted to speak with the victims first to check in and talk with them. I called the main office to see if they could call them out of class, one at a time. Within five minutes, I had all five outside my office. I guess the "one at at time" was not understood very well. I stuck my head out of the door and introduced myself.

I asked them if they wanted to see me individually or all together. They all walked in. Well, that answered my question. I did not have enough seats in my office and was about to go get a few more chairs when three of them sat on the floor. They said they did not need the chairs but thanked me for the thought. I closed the door. I asked them if they had an idea of why they were there and one of them held out his phone. He told me to have a look at it. I began to scroll down the messages and saw very similar comments that were on Michelle's phone. I asked if others had similar comments and the other four held out their phones for me to see. I walked around to each of them and quickly scrolled their phones. Almost identical comments, each spewing such hatred. My stomach turned as I made my way back to my desk. I asked them if they knew the people who had started this and they all said, almost in unison, the names of all four girls involved. I then asked if any of them had talked to their parents or someone about what was going on and each of them had. I was informed that these were the parents who had contacted the school last year. This made things a bit easier, as all parents were in the know. I asked each of the students to text their parents and see if they were available to go on a speaker call with me. They all agreed. Each parent was called and placed on speaker, and I began the conversation:

Hey everyone. My name is Constable Sheremata, and I am the School Resource Officer here at the high school. Thank you for each taking a few minutes out of your day to come on the call. I have each of your kids here in my office talking with me about a bullying issue that had started last year. It seems to be getting worse and I want to get it dealt with ASAP before it takes another terrible turn. I have already spoken with the principal from last year, so I have some information. I do have a request though, and I will need permission from you parents. May I have your kids' cell phones for the rest of today and they can come and pick them up tomorrow? I would like to get screen shots of the comments and be able to scroll through all the messages and comments that your kids have had to deal with. None of your kids are in trouble and I will not be checking their phones for any other information. You have my word. If you are okay with that, can each of you say your name and your kid's name? Also, could you each text your kids' phone with a confirmation of that. I want to make sure we are all on the same page. If you have any further questions or concerns, I will give your kids my number and you can reach out at any time. Do any of you have any questions? If not thank you again so much for taking the time for my call. I will get to the bottom of this and make sure your kids will not have to continue living with this torment.

I looked at all the kids as their parents each agreed and said goodbye. I asked each of them if the phone thing was okay and they all nodded. One of them even said it would be a breath of fresh air not having it. I thanked all the students for coming down and I told them that they had my word that I would do everything I could to resolve this. As each of them got up, they handed me their phone and one by one gave me a hug. Wow, I was not expecting that. It warmed my heart. I knew I had a lot of work ahead of me, but I needed to get to the bottom of this. I did not want someone else to take their life.

As soon as the students left, I began to look through each phone and saw the comments and messages that were continuing to pop up. I got the names of the four girls who were the main offenders and went to the principal's office. I let her know where I was at with the investigation and asked if she would be present when I spoke with each of these girls. She agreed. I had the office secretary call down the first girl, JB. She was the one with the least number of messages and comments sent. She arrived in the main office within five minutes of my calling her down. The principal went and got her while I sat and waited in the principal's office. Both the principal and JB walked in, and she was surprised to see me. At that moment, I saw her face change and it was as if she knew she had been caught. I introduced myself to her, asked her to please place her phone on the desk, and asked her if she knew why she was there. I noticed she began to fidget with her hands, and she was kicking her feet back and forth. She looked at me and quietly whispered, "Yes." I asked her to explain. JB began her story:

> I believe it's because I and three other girls have been sending nasty messages and comments to other students. I did not want to hurt anybody, and I did it because I thought it was a joke. I had joined the group last, and I had been so excited that these girls had allowed me into their circle. Then when I found out about John, I knew it was not a joke anymore.

I asked JB how telling someone to kill themselves and that the school would be a better place without them sounded like a joke. That was the furthest thing from a joke. I asked her who the other girls were. She saw that I had a bunch of phones and realized the jig was up. She broke down crying and gave me the names. AG, BB, and the leader was DL. I thanked her for being upfront and honest. I also let her know that I would be contacting her parents and inform them of what had transpired over these past couple of years. She nodded her head. I asked the principal to move her into another office so the other girls would not see her here and that I would be keeping her phone until her parents came. I then had AG called down. The principal went out and got her from the front, and as soon as she walked into the principal's office and saw me, she tried to run out the door. I stopped her and asked her why she was trying to run. She said it was not her fault. I asked her to sit down, place her cell phone on the desk, and explain what she meant. She informed me that DL was the head of the group and her and DL had been friends since grade six. She said that DL could be a nice person, but she also had this mean streak that would come over her. I asked her what that meant. AG explained:

> *DL would be nice to you if you did as she said or gave her things. As soon as you disagree with her, watch out. She would make your life miserable. If someone got a better mark than her, or got the lead in a school play, she would start to torment them by spreading rumors and sending nasty messages and comments throughout social media about them. She would bully people into doing what she wanted. I remember that another girl who was part of the group, BB, and I were friends first in grade three. We were inseparable. We always hung out. Then in grade six DL arrived at the school and there was something about her that BB did not like so she told me to be careful. DL found out about what BB had said and for all of grade six, DL bullied BB, making her life miserable. BB did not even want to come to school. Then in grade seven, DL*

got caught shoplifting and BB took the fall for her. So now, BB was in DL's good books and welcomed into the group. Now as I'm talking about it, it sounds so messed up. The three of us would hang out, and if DL did not like someone, she would start rumors about them and both BB and I would follow her. JB came to the school I think in later part of grade eight. DL did not like her right off the bat because JB was way prettier than DL. So doing what DL did best, she began to start rumors about JB sleeping around and how she was a slut. Well, that backfired because many people knew JB as she was a part of many community groups and they also knew that she went to church and did not sleep around, so to save face, DL invited her to become a part of our group. Again, how messed up was that? Constable S, I'm going to be honest here, as I hear myself talking and explaining to you all about this so-called "friend" group, I cannot believe I ever allowed myself to become a part of this. I am so embarrassed. I deserve whatever is coming.

AG placed her face in her hands and began to cry. I handed her a Kleenex and thanked her for being so honest. I let her know that I would be calling her parents to let them know about all that had been happening. I told her that I would keep her phone until her parents came down and then asked her to sit in another office while the next girl came down. I wanted to talk with the ringleader, DL next. I wondered if she was going to be as upfront and honest or if she was going to blame someone else. I asked the secretary to call her down. The principal and I were ready. The principal went out to get her from the office. They both walked into the principal's office and as DL saw me, she gave a little smirk. "So, who ratted me out? You cannot prove anything." Wow, I was not expecting that at all. We were now dealing with a very narcissistic youth who always had to have control of the situation. This was going to be interesting. I asked her to sit down and then introduced myself to her. I also asked her to please place her cell phone on the desk. She slammed the phone down on the desk. DL couldn't have cared less who I was. She began to ask if it was AG, BB, or JB that told on her. I told her none of the above. I brought out all the phones I had from the victims, and her face turned white. She knew that she had been caught. "DL," I said, "this can go a couple of ways. You can either be honest about everything that has happened, and we can have a conversation, or you are not honest, and we don't have a conversation. It's your call. The truth will be way easier in the long run." She looked at me and said, "I'll tell you the truth and I will talk." She began her story:

> I have always had a hard time fitting in and so I learned at an early age that I could control situations quite easily and I began to use that to my advantage. In grade six I came to the school that AG and BB were at. I did not know anyone, and AG came over and was friendly to me. Then I met her friend BB, and I did not like her because she did not trust me. She would tell AG to stay away from me. So, I began to say mean things about her so people would not like her. That worked for a while. Then in grade seven, I got caught shoplifting and I told BB that she better take the fall for me, and if she did then she could come into our group. So she did, and I let her in the group. Then in grade eight, I believe, JB came to the school. I hated her because she was gorgeous and all the boys wanted to be with her. I did

what I was good at and started a bunch of rumors. Well, that did not go well for me. It kind of backfired on me so I invited her into the group instead. Then, in grade nine, one of the girls, Michelle, got an award that I should have received, and she was also picked over me for a main part in the school play, and I could not have that. I began to send messages and comments all over social media about her, including telling her to kill herself. I hated her. That worked so well for me that I started picking out students that had things going for them and started rumors and saying things on social media. It made me feel so good to see these others hurting. You probably heard about John. I did not make him kill himself. He chose to do that. I may have said some mean things, but I am not to blame for his death. I have a lot of hate inside and when I hurt people, I feel better. That's who I am.

Well, I got my answers. I was just not expecting her to be that honest. She was a hurting little girl with so much pain inside. I thanked her for telling me the truth and I told her that I was going to be contacting her parents and updating them on everything that was learned today. I also said I would be keeping her phone until her parents came to get her. The principal then spoke up and let her know that with all the information that had come forward, she would be suspending DL and possibly be looking at further consequences. The saddest thing with all of this was that DL felt no remorse. How could a fifteen-year-old feel nothing about the pain that she had caused so many people?

I had DL stay in the principal's office while the principal and I went out to talk about our plan of action. I was going to contact

DL's parents first and then contact the other parents. I went back to where DL was and asked for her parents' number. She sat there emotionless and gave me their number. I called and spoke with her mom. I asked if both her mom and dad could come to the school, as we had a major situation that we were dealing with. DL's mom said they would be there in about ten minutes. Perfect. One down, three more to go. I had DL stay in that office and I went over to the next one where JB was. I asked her for her parents' number, and I called them to ask them both to come to the school as a situation had occurred with their daughter. They were on their way. I then went to see AG and had her give me her parents' number. I called them, let them know we had a situation with their daughter and if they could come to the school. They were also on their way. The only one who had not been talked with was BB. She was sitting in the main office as she had been called down. I motioned for her to come into the lounge area as there were no more available offices. I let her know what had transpired and this young girl fell to her knees, sobbing. Through her sobs, she said she was so sorry and that she had not wanted to be a part of things but was so terrified of DL. She was so thankful that this was the end of it. I gave her a Kleenex and let her know I was going to call her parents as they needed to know what had been going on. She agreed and gave me their number. I called them and they were heading to the school. Now came the hard part: watching how each of these parents would react with what they would be finding out. AG's parents got to the school first and I had them come into the office where AG was. I introduced myself and informed them about what had all transpired. AG's mom shook her head and her dad looked at her and told her they had warned her about DL. They thought there was something off with her. AG's mom told AG that she would not have her cell phone for the rest of the semester, and they would then talk about the next semester. They also told AG that they expected her to write a letter to each of the students that had been affected and apologize to them. Her mom looked at me with such shame. She told me that this was not how they raised AG. I let AG and her parents know that she was suspended for three days, and after that, she was to come back for a meeting with the principal and myself. Her parents thanked me and made their way with AG out of the main office.

Next was BB. I brought her parents into the lounge area and told them what all had happened and how BB was involved. I let them know that BB was very remorseful. Her parents informed her that her phone and going out privileges were gone and that she was to write an apology letter to each of the victims. BB said she would. I could see relief come over BB's whole body. I also let BB know that she was suspended for three days and then was to come back with her parents for a meeting with the principal and myself.

JB's mom came next. Her dad was away for work. I informed her mom about everything that had come out this afternoon. JB sat looking at her mom with such shame and sadness. Her mom took her phone away and told her she would not be needing it for a while. Then she told JB that she would write an apology letter to each victim. JB's mom could not believe that her daughter could do something like this. She would be letting JB's father know as soon as they left. I also informed JB that she was suspended from school for three days and she was to come back with her parents for a meeting with me and the principal afterward. She nodded. Her mom thanked me, shook my hand, and took JB out the door. Three out of the way and one more to go. I went out to the main office area and saw a couple sitting out there. I asked if they were DL's parents. They said yes. They then asked how bad things were. Now that was a different type of question. I brought them back to the principal's office. Both the principal and I stood and the three of them sat down. I told DL's parents what had all transpired, and I included everything from grade nine and on. Both parents just shook their heads, her mom had tears welling up in her eyes. When I finished, her dad looked at her phone on the desk and told her that he was taking that back, as well all social media accounts would be taken down and computer use at home was for schoolwork only. The principal then let them know that DL would be suspended for five days and then was to come back with her parents for a meeting with both me and the principal. DL was informed that she could be looking at expulsion. DL sat emotionless. Her parents looked so sad. They then asked about the victims and how they were doing. I let them know that I was working with them, and they were going to be okay, but it was going to take time. Her parents told me that they were going to get her to write an apology to the people that were affected. DL yelled, "Over my dead body will I do that!" I looked at the principal and I knew she was thinking the same thing I was. That just made the decision for expulsion way easier. Before DL got up to leave, I informed her that I was looking into filing charges, as what she had done was not okay and there were consequences for her actions. I was going to be meeting with my supervisor to go through the case and I would know more when she came back in five days for her meeting. She was not to have any contact with any of the girls or victims for right now. DL and her parents walked out the door. Both her mom and dad turned around, shook my and the principal's hands, and said they were so sorry. My heart felt for them. That was not an easy situation.

I looked at the time and realized it had only been half a day. A lot sure had happened. I thanked the principal and told her I needed all the victims back in my office. I wanted to let them know that things were on the mend. The office staff had them come to my office, and as I made my way back to my office, I felt a little skip in my step. It felt kind of nice, as it had been such a heavy morning. As I unlocked the door to my office, the students arrived, and I had them all come in. They sat down and I let them know that the bullying had now stopped, the offenders had been dealt with, and now came the healing process. This would take time but that was okay.

I asked if I could keep their phones until tomorrow, as I wanted to get all the evidence that I needed to work on this case, but I asked if they would each put their parents on speaker phone so I could update them all at once. Once all the parents were on speaker, I let them all know that the offenders had been dealt with and I was continuing to gather evidence as there may be possible charges still coming.

I asked that each of the parents support their kids through this long healing process and to seek someone to talk with and meet with. I thanked them for trusting me with this situation and that if they wanted to come in and meet with me, they could. The students all ended the calls on their phones, placed them back on my desk, and all came in for a group hug. What a feeling. I had tears in my eyes. The students left and then it was time for all the paperwork. Never a dull day in high school.

Bullying is not just an issue for those directly involved; it reverberates through entire communities, impacting everyone from victims to bystanders, and even the bullies themselves. As you reflect on this story and information shared, it's crucial to recognize all our collective responsibility in addressing and preventing bullying. By showing empathy and awareness, by being an active bystander, by building strong support systems, and educating ourselves, and advocating for others, we can take these vital steps toward long-term change. Remember, creating a compassionate and supportive community begins with each of us. By standing up against bullying, we can help ensure a safer, kinder world for everyone.

CHAPTER 10

Final Say with Carlamay

As we draw this journey to a close, it's clear that the landscape of teenage life is as complex as it is profound. The issues we've discussed—suicide, eating disorders, bullying, domestic abuse, and substance abuse to name a few—are stark reminders of the challenges that today's youth face. These are not just isolated problems; they are interconnected struggles that weave through the daily lives of young people. Yet, amidst these challenges, there is hope. This hope lies in our ability to have meaningful conversations that offer support, understanding, and empowerment.

The Power of Listening

Throughout this book, we've seen how crucial it is to truly listen to the voices of youth. Listening is more than just hearing words; it's about understanding the emotions and experiences that those words represent. When we listen with our hearts, we create a safe space where youth feel valued and understood. This is the foundation of any meaningful conversation and the first step towards healing and empowerment.

Creating Safe Spaces

One of the most important lessons we've learned is the significance of creating safe spaces for youth to express themselves. Whether it's at home, in schools, or within the community, these environments must be free from judgment and full of compassion. Youths need to know that their feelings are valid and that there is always someone willing to listen and help them navigate their struggles.

Honest and Open Conversations

Having honest and open conversations about difficult topics is not easy, but it is essential. These discussions can be uncomfortable, but they are necessary to break down the walls of silence and stigma that often surround issues like suicide, eating disorders, and substance abuse. By addressing these topics head-on, we can provide youth with the tools and support they need to cope and thrive.

Empathy and Compassion

Empathy and compassion are the cornerstones of impactful communication. When we approach youth with empathy, we acknowledge their pain and struggles without minimizing their experiences. Compassion drives us to take action, offering support and resources that can make a real difference in their lives.

Empowering Youth

Empowerment comes from giving youth a voice and validating their experiences. It means involving them in conversations about their lives and decisions affecting them. By empowering youth, we help them build confidence and resilience, enabling them to overcome obstacles and pursue their dreams.

The Role of Community

It takes a village to raise a child, and this adage holds true in addressing the issues facing today's youth. Schools, families, friends, and community organizations all play a pivotal role in supporting youth. Collaborative efforts can create a network of support that ensures no youth feels alone in their struggles.

A Call to Action

As we close this chapter, let us remember that the journey does not end here. The insights and stories shared in this book are just the beginning. It is now up to each of us to take action. We must commit to being present, to listening, and to having those tough conversations that can change lives.

If you are a parent, teacher, mentor, or friend, your role is vital. Approach the youth in your life with an open heart and a willingness to listen. Educate yourself about the issues they face and be proactive in offering support. Your actions can provide the foundation for a brighter future for the youth you care about.

For the young people reading this book, know that your voice matters. Your experiences and feelings are valid. Do not be afraid to reach out for help or to speak your truth. There are people who care deeply about you and want to help you navigate the challenges you face.

Conclusion

The journey through the truths of young life is one filled with both challenges and opportunities. By fostering open, honest, and compassionate conversations, we can help youths feel seen, heard, and valued. Together, we can create a world where young people are empowered to face their struggles with confidence and resilience, knowing they are not alone.

Let us move forward with a heart for youth, committed to making a difference one conversation at a time. The future is bright, and it begins with us.

Gratitude and Appreciation

Writing this book has been a journey filled with learning, challenges and growth. I am deeply grateful to the many people who have supported and inspired me throughout this process.

First and foremost, I want to thank my Lord and Savior, Jesus Christ, for giving me the creative mind, the empathy and compassion for others, the gifts of serving and discernment that have allowed me to bring this book together.

Thank you to my husband, Michael, for your unwavering love, encouragement, and belief in me. Your support has been invaluable as you walked beside me through the blood, sweat and tears as I wrote this book.

Thank you to my son Jackson for being the rock when some days I felt that life was getting away from me. We never know what life will throw our way and your resilience has been unbelievable. I am so blessed that God gave you to me and that I get to be your momma!

Thank you to my mom and dad, Lorraine and Lorey, for all your love and support as I grew up. Thank you for always allowing me to be myself and to shine in ways that others could not always understand, but you did!

Thank you to my brother Kyle (KC), for always being a support no matter where you were in the world. Life has not always been wine and roses, but together, we have made it to be such an amazing journey. I knew that day long ago, God was not done with you yet. You had so much more living to do and I am so thankful that we have gotten to grow together!

Thank you to Darity Wesley and the whole Steve Harrison Team for your expertise and dedication. Darity, you were that push that I needed, that one person who knew I could get it done! Your insights and hard work have significantly shaped this book and brought it to life.

Thank you to each of my first readers for taking time out of your busy schedules to read through the manuscript and give me your honest, heartfelt feedback. Norma Omichinski, Connie Jakab, Kristine Davis, David Savage, Bret Ridgway, and Carolee Turner, thank you from the bottom of my heart for your input, critiquing and honesty when it came to such deep topics.

Lastly, I want to express my heartfelt thanks to my readers. Your interest and engagement are what make this journey worthwhile. I hope this book resonates with you and provides value in your lives.

With greatest gratitude.

Carlamay Sheremata

Resources

Emergency: If you need immediate assistance because someone is in danger or hurting him or herself or someone else, then call the police. Call: 911

Kids Help Phone: 24/7 mental health service offering free, confidential support to young people
In Canada Call: 1-800-668-6868
In the United States text: HOME to 741741

Distress Centre (Calgary, Canada): 24/7 crisis line via phone or chat
Call: 1-403-266-HELP (4357)
In the United States Call or Text: 988

Calgary Pregnancy Care Centre: Pregnancy and family support
Call: 1-403-269-3110

National Child Abuse Hotline: 24/7 help if you have been sexually and physically abused.
In the United States Call:1-800-422-4453

Alcohol and Drug Abuse Hotline: 24/7
In the United States Call: 1-800-821-4357

Domestic Violence and Abuse Hotline
In Calgary 1-866-606 SAFE (7233)
In the United States 1-800-799-SAFE (7233)

About the Author

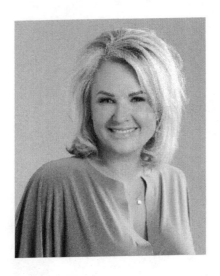

Carlamay Sheremata is a retired police officer who resides in Calgary, Alberta, Canada. For the last twenty-one years, she has had extensive experience in school environments fostering positive relationships with both students and staff, specialized training in adolescent development, along with extensive mental health training which has enabled her to effectively communicate and engage with students of all ages, addressing their unique needs and concerns. Carlamay has been a part of numerous media interviews and has appeared on several television broadcasts. Drawing on her extensive experience in law enforcement, Carlamay brings a unique perspective to her writing. She focuses on the resilience and strength of individuals facing adversity.

Deeply passionate about the well-being of youth, Carlamay believes that young people today face significant challenges and are yearning to be heard with grace, love, and compassion. She advocates for giving young people a voice, recognizing their potential and the importance of listening to their experiences and perspectives. Carlamay's commitment to empowering the next generation is a central theme in her writing and personal philosophy.

When she's not writing, Carlamay enjoys singing, serving others, and cherishing time with her husband and son, along with other family and friends. She is dedicated to creating a lasting legacy through her work and personal life.

Work with Carlamay

Carlamay Sheremata is available for podcasts,
speaking engagements and workshops.

She also provides one-on-one and group coaching,
plus tools and resources for leading
Youth Truth conversations.

Contact her at **www.carlamaysheremata.com**

Manufactured by Amazon.ca
Bolton, ON